T0201352

Microneedling

Microneedling

Global Perspectives in Aesthetic Medicine

Edited by

Elizabeth Bahar Houshmand

Series Editor

Michael H. Gold

WILEY Blackwell

Registered Offices
John Wiley & Sons, Inc., 111 River Street, Hoboken, NJ 07030, USA
John Wiley & Sons Ltd, The Atrium, Southern Gate, Chichester, West Sussex, PO19 8SQ, UK

Editorial Office
9600 Garsington Road, Oxford, OX4 2DQ, UK

For details of our global editorial offices, customer services, and more information about Wiley products visit us at www.wiley.com.

Wiley also publishes its books in a variety of electronic formats and by print-on-demand. Some content that appears in standard print versions of this book may not be available in other formats.

Library of Congress Cataloging-in-Publication Data
Name: Houshmand, Elizabeth Bahar, editor.
Title: Microneedling : global perspectives in aesthetic medicine / edited
    by Elizabeth Bahar Houshmand.
Other titles: Cosmetic and aesthetic dermatology series.
Description: Hoboken, NJ : John Wiley & Sons, Inc., 2021. | Series:
    Cosmetic and aesthetic dermatology series | Includes bibliographical
    references and index.
Identifiers: LCCN 2020055815 (print) | LCCN 2020055816 (ebook) | ISBN
    9781119431923 (cloth) | ISBN 9781119431831 (adobe pdf) | ISBN
    9781119431947 (epub)
Subjects: MESH: Skin Diseases–therapy | Cosmetic Techniques | Minimally
    Invasive Surgical Procedures–instrumentation | Needles
Classification: LCC RD119 (print) | LCC RD119 (ebook) | NLM WR 650 | DDC
    617.9/5–dc23
LC record available at https://lccn.loc.gov/2020055815
LC ebook record available at https://lccn.loc.gov/2020055816

Cover Design: Wiley
Cover Image: © Mark Nazh/Shutterstock.com

Set in 10/12.5pt MinionPro by SPi Global, Pondicherry, India

Printed in Great Britain by Bell and Bain Ltd, Glasgow

10 9 8 7 6 5 4 3 2 1

Contents

List of Editors and Contributors

Michael H. Gold, MD
Gold Skin Care Center
Tennessee Clinical Research Center
Nashville, TN, USA

Elizabeth Bahar Houshmand, MD, FAAD, FABIM
Houshmand Dermatology and Wellness
Dallas, TX, USA

Atchima Suwanchinda, MD, MSc
School of Anti-aging and Regenerative
Medicine, Mae Fah Luang University
Ramathibodi University Hospital,
Mahidol University
Bangkok, Thailand

Chytra V. Anand, MD
Kosmoderma Clinics
Bangalore, India

Desmond Fernandes, MB, BCh, FRCS (Edin)
Department of Plastic and Reconstructive Surgery
Faculty of Medicine
University of Cape Town

Matthias Aust, MD
Aust Aesthetik
Landsberg am Lech, Germany

Parinitha Rao, MBBS, MD
Kosmoderma Clinics
Bangalore, India

Richard Bender, MD
St. Vinzenz Hospital Cologne Plastische Chirurgie
Cologne, Germany

Stuti Khare Shukla, MD
Elements of Aesthetics Clinics
Dr. Stuti Khare's Skin & Hair Clinics
Mumbai, India

Cosmetic and Aesthetic Procedures in Dermatology Series

The scope and field of cosmetic surgery have changed and grown over the past decade. We have a myriad of new and exciting noninvasive or minimally invasive techniques and treatments that have helped propel this growth. With injectables, energy-based devices, and skincare, we now have the tools at our disposal to reverse signs of aging and to successfully treat cosmetic concerns with minimal downtime and with outstanding clinical results.

Several years ago, we began discussing the idea of producing a series of cosmetic dermatology textbooks edited by masters in their fields and written by some of the best minds in our discipline. While it is not always easy to get these kinds of projects off the ground, we are pleased that with persistence and great guidance from the Wiley teams, we are now able to present an entire series on the various aspects of cosmetic dermatology.

Through this textbook series on cosmetic and aesthetic dermatology, clinicians will have the tools available to help treat patients with the most advanced techniques and with the most appropriate guidance that has been presented to date. Each volume in this series has been meticulously thought out; each is edited by one of the most significant thought leaders in our field, and each chapter will bring to life this incredible field we live in, and illuminate how we are able to transform lives and make our patients better.

We hope you enjoy this series of books as they are rolled out. It is our joy and pleasure to bring them to you.

Michael H. Gold, MD
Series Editor

Preface

The skin is our canvas. As a board certified dermatologist, it is my mission to help all my patients achieve healthy, beautiful skin. Through education, teaching, and research this is possible. This textbook is a continuation of this mission, inspired by the drive to create the best possible outcomes for my patients, and the love of being a physician and educator.

Over the last several years, minimally invasive procedures have significantly increased in the worlds of dermatology, plastic surgery, and aesthetic medicine. This textbook is a global consortium of the leaders in these fields and experts on microneedling.

Microneedling is an outstanding option for patients of all skin types and ethnicities who desire measurable clinical results from treatments with little to no downtime. It is a relatively new option in dermatology and has been utilized for a broad range of applications, including skin rejuvenation, acne scarring, rhytides, surgical scars, dyschromia, melasma, enlarged pores, and transdermal drug delivery.

Microneedling is a safe, minimally invasive, and effective aesthetic treatment for several different dermatologic conditions. Given its expedient post-treatment recovery, minimal side effect profile, and significant clinical results, microneedling is a valuable alternative to more invasive procedures. The chapters of this book discuss the various applications in detail.

I want to thank my family and mentors for their support always. I also want to give a special thank-you to Dr. Michael Gold. He is an innovator in our field and I am happy to call him my dear friend, mentor, and colleague.

Elizabeth Bahar Houshmand, M.D.
Diplomat American Board of Dermatology
Diplomat American Board of Internal Medicine
Fellow American Society of Laser Medicine
Instagram: @HoushmandMD
Website: Houshmanddermatology.com

1

Introduction to Microneedling

Elizabeth Bahar Houshmand

Houshmand Dermatology and Wellness, Dallas, TX, USA

Introduction

Microneedling is a minimally invasive procedure that uses fine needles to puncture the epidermis. The microwounds created stimulate the release of growth factors and induce collagen production. The epidermis remains relatively intact during the procedure.

Microneedling initially was utilized as a collagen induction therapy for facial scars and skin rejuvenation, but it is now widely used for multiple indications, including transdermal delivery system for therapeutic drugs and in combination therapies. The indications for microneedling have grown as research and clinical applications have expanded widely in dermatology and dermatologic surgery.

In this textbook, the authors highlight the constantly evolving research and developments in microneedling techniques and instruments, along with microneedling's applications in dermatology and aesthetic medicine. We are honored to provide a comprehensive and global perspective from key opinion leaders in dermatology and plastic surgery from around the world.

History

Microneedling, or percutaneous collagen induction therapy, was introduced in the 1990s for the treatment of scars, striae, and laxity [1]. The use of needles for non-ablative skin treatment was first described by Orentreich and Orentreich in 1995

Microneedling: Global Perspectives in Aesthetic Medicine, First Edition.
Edited by Elizabeth Bahar Houshmand.
© 2021 John Wiley & Sons Ltd. Published 2021 by John Wiley & Sons Ltd.

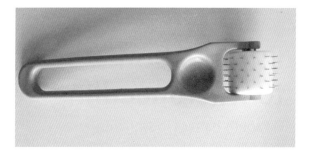

Figure 1.1 Original microneedling roller created by Dr. Desmond Fernandes in 2001. Fixed needle length of 3.0 mm multiuse roller; designed for reuse on a single patient for approximately six treatment sessions. The original rollers were not able to be autoclaved at that time. They were sterilized by soaking in instrument cleaning fluid. *Source:* Dr. Desmond Fernandes.

as subcision surgery, which is the release of depressed scars and wrinkles with a needle from their attachment to the underlying skin. This controlled trauma leads to the formation of connective tissue to fill the created gap.

In 1996, skin needling using a roller device was introduced by Fernandes at the International Society of Aesthetic Plastic Surgery (ISAPS) congress in Taipei [2]. In 1997, Camirand and Doucet introduced dry tattooing without pigment as needle dermabrasion and proposed it as a technique to improve the appearance of scars [3].

Fernandes, in 2001, developed the original percutaneous collage induction dermaroller with needles. His pilot roller device was a drum-shaped tool, with a cylinder and 3 mm needles that reach the fibroblasts deep in the reticular layer (see Figure 1.1).

Zeitter et al. confirmed Fernandes's findings and made a modified roller. They concluded that 1 mm needles show similar results to 3 mm needles, with the advantage of less downtime, swelling, and pain [3, 4].

Mechanism of action

The mechanism of action is thought to be a disruption of the epidermis and dermis. Micropunctures are created using microneedles, which produce a controlled skin injury without damaging the epidermis. The mechanical microinjury results in the classic wound-healing cascade and stimulates cellular proliferation and migration through the stimulation of growth factors (see Figure 1.2).

These microinjuries lead to minimal superficial bleeding and set up a wound-healing cascade with release of various growth factors, such as platelet-derived growth factor (PDGF), transforming growth factor alpha and beta (TGFα and TGFβ), connective tissue activating protein, connective tissue growth factor, and fibroblast growth factor (FGF) [5]. The needles also break down the scar strands

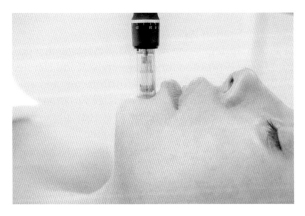

Figure 1.2 The electric pen-shaped device has adjustable settings to control the speed and depth of needle penetration. *Source:* skvalval/Shutterstock.

and allow them to revascularize. Neovascularization and neocollagenesis are initiated by migration and proliferation of fibroblasts and laying down of an intercellular matrix [6, 7]. A fibronectin matrix forms five days after injury and determines the deposition of collagen, resulting in skin tightening persisting for five to seven years in the form of collagen III. The depth of neocollagenesis has been found to be 5–600 μm with a 1.5 mm length needle. Histological examination of the skin treated with four microneedling sessions one month apart shows up to 400% increase in collagen and elastin deposition at six months postoperatively, with a thickened stratum spinosum and normal rete ridges at one year postoperatively [8]. Collagen fiber bundles appear to have a normal lattice pattern rather than parallel bundles as in scar tissue [9].

The devices used create transient epidermal and dermal openings ranging in size from 25 to 3000 um in depth as a microinjury, with the goal of stimulating the inherent skin repair mechanisms. These microwounds or microinjuries initiate the release of growth factors, which trigger and stimulate collagen and elastin formation in the dermis. That leads to healthier skin with improved texture. The microwounds are microchannels and heal following the classic wound-healing cascade: inflammation, proliferation, and remodeling. This cascade is brought on by the needles' disruption of the stratum corneum; the endothelial lining and the subendothelial matrix recruits platelets and neutrophils to the site of injury. Needling exposes thrombin and collagen fragments, which attract and activate platelets. The platelets form a plug and initiate the clotting cascade, which involves local platelet aggregation, inflammation, and blood coagulation through increased levels of thrombin and fibrin.

The needles carry an electric potential that stimulates fibroblast proliferation [10]. The mechanical injury triggers the release of potassium and proteins that alter intercellular resting potential, drawing in fibroblasts and stimulating neocollagenesis and revascularization [6].

Research has shown up-regulation of TGFβ3, a cytokine that prevents aberrant scarring; increased gene expression for collagen type I; and elevated levels of vascular endothelial growth factor, fibroblast growth factor, and epidermal growth factor [11–13]. Histological studies have shown huge variation in epidermal thickness. Randomized murine studies have reported statistically significant epidermal thickening from 140% up to 685% after microneedling plus topical vitamins A and C when compared to control [13, 14]. This is thought to be one of the reasons microneedling is effective for scar therapy and notable skin rejuvenation.

A human study of 480 patients treated with microneedling plus topical vitamins A and C reported thickening of the stratum spinosum lasting up to one year [8, 15].

Increased collagen types I, III, and VII and tropoelastin in human biopsies were found after six sessions of microneedling, ten with elevated levels of collagen type I and elastin persisting at six months. The number of melanocytes was unchanged postprocedurally.

These results support the safe use of this modality in patients with darker skin types [8, 15]. Having a safe and effective treatment modality for all skin types is advantageous in an aesthetic practice.

The devices

Modern microneedling devices consist of rollers, stamps, and pens. Needling devices have evolved over the past decade through a variety of advancements. Currently, there are multiple devices based on needle length, drum size, and automation. To date, there are five FDA-approved pen devices. Physicians and providers need to consider important factors like needle length, needle material, and clinical indications in selecting which device to utilize [9].

Pens

Most pens utilize sterile single-use cartridges and variable needle length to be able to customize the treatment depending on the unique characteristics of the patient's skin and the area being treated. They are automated and the physician has the ability to adjust the needle length for customized treatment options and the pressure and depth during treatment can be more uniform (see Figure 1.3) [16].

The pen itself is reusable, and most pens have a protective disposable sleeve. The needle tips are the disposable/consumable in these devices. Because of their size the tips are able to treat curved and small areas such as the nasal ala and the

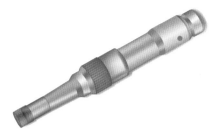

Figure 1.3 Pen: Single-use cartridge with adjustable frequency and needle length. *Source:* Sakurra/Shutterstock.

periocular and perioral areas. Most devices have a rechargeable battery that operates in two modes: high speed mode (700 cycles/minute) and low speed mode (412 cycles/minute) in a vibrating stamplike manner [17].

The devices contain multiple fine needles, ranging from 0.5 to 1.5 mm in length, that are rolled onto the skin. Needles between 1.5 and 3.0 mm are available but are preferred for the use of scars and damaged skin. The roller device is a drum-shaped tool with a cylindrical head that is rolled back and forth to induce thousands of tiny pores in the stratum corneum and papillary dermis.

The length of needle selected for an individual patient depends upon the indication for microneedling and on the thickness of epidermis and dermis of the skin being treated. For treating acne and other scars, on average a needle length of 1.5–2 mm is utilized. When microneedling is used as a procedure to treat skin aging and wrinkles, a needle length of 0.5 mm or 1.0 mm is recommended [18]. The frequency interval for microneedling depends upon the indication for which the procedure is being done as well as the needle length of the dermaroller device used. Microneedling generally requires more than one session and a series of treatments is usually recommended.

Five basic types of medical dermarollers, which are registered with the FDA, have been described in the dermaroller series by Anastassakis and most dermarolling devices are adopted from these elementary types [19].

Stamps

Stamps were popular in the late 1990s and have made a resurgence recently. The stamps currently offered have attached microchambers which have the ability to directly administer a form of mesotherapy using the stamping device. Stamps have different needle lengths (0.2–3 mm) and a diameter of 0.12 mm These are useful in the administration of treatment to scars and anatomically small surface areas such as the perioral, periocular, and nasal regions where greater control is beneficial, and may be used on isolated scars and wrinkles (see Figure 1.4) [3, 20–22].

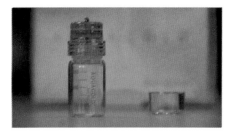

Figure 1.4 Microneedling stamp: fixed needle length with customizable vial for needling infusion. *Source:* Aquavit Pharmaceuticals, Inc.

Rollers

Rollers have many fine-gauged needles that are on a cylindrical surface that pierces the skin on an angle. The rollers are fixed; the parameters are uniform for each device that you use. Unlike pens, you can not mechanically adjust rollers. The quality of rollers is also critical. Patients are seeking at-home rollers but the quality of the needles is paramount. Needles that are dull or loose may cause tears in the skin and foreign body reactions, including but not limited to granulomas.

The most important factor is needle length. A high ratio of tip length to diameter (13:1) is an important property of good needles [9]. The length of needle selected for an individual patient depends upon the indication for microneedling. For treating acne and other scars as a routine, a needle length of 1.5–2 mm is usually used. When microneedling is used as a procedure to treat aging skin and wrinkles, a needle length of 0.5 mm or 1.0 mm is usually recommended [19]. The needle length to use will also depend on the thickness of the epidermis and dermis of the skin for optimal results.

Given their design and mechanics, rollers are able to pierce the skin deeper when at a 90-degree angle or perpendicular to the skin. Fernandes showed that with the use of rollers you have an intact epidermis with microchannels spaced out with about a four-cell width distribution [4]. The provider's technique with these devices is critical. Tearing of the epidermis may occur if performed incorrectly, with too much pressure, or at an increased speed. The needle rollers themselves are variable based on the materials used, needle length and diameter, and total number of needles. The quality of the rollers is also critical to evaluate.

Needle length is generally 0.2–3.00 mm, with a diameter of > 0.25mm and the materials are variable: stainless steel, titanium, or silver and gold. Stainless steel is the most common type of needle, silver and gold offer antimicrobial properties and carry less of a risk of allergic reactions, and titanium needles usually stay sharper longer (see Figure 1.5).

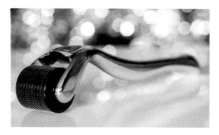

Figure 1.5 Current rollers with fixed needle length; some current models are autoclavable. *Source:* marcinm111/Shutterstock.

DermaFrac

DermaFrac treatment is a newer modification of microneedling combining microdermabrasion, microneedling, simultaneous deep tissue serum infusion, and light emitting diode (LED) therapy. DermaFrac treatments target aging and sun damaged skin, acne, enlarged pores, uneven skin tone, wrinkles, fine lines, hyperpigmentation, and superficial scars. It takes approximately 45 minutes to complete a full face treatment when all four modalities are used. This noninvasive, cost-effective treatment carries the advantage of having no downtime, with individualized selection of serums for infusion (see Figure 1.6) [22].

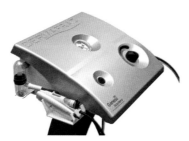

Figure 1.6 DermaFrac™: Microneedling device combining simultaneous customized infusion followed by LED light therapy. *Source:* Genesis Biosystems, Inc.

Clinical considerations

Microneedling is not only used for rejuvenation of the skin. Its use in dermatology and aesthetic medicine has expanded to include the treatment of acne scars, alopecia, dyspigmentation, alopecia, striae, and for many other indications. It can be utilized alone or in combination with other treatment modalities, such as chemical peels, platelet-rich plasma, radiofrequency, subcision, punch elevation, and lasers. It is often used in conjunction with a topical formulation to enhance its penetration and action.

Microneedling is safely used for enhanced drug delivery to the deeper epidermis and dermis by bypassing the stratum corneum. This strategy has been utilized for burn patients and for rejuvenation, allowing cosmeceuticals to be delivered more deeply. Caution is necessary in deciding which topicals to use during delivery, as inflammation may occur and granulomas have been noted.

Conclusion

Microneedling is a popular treatment in dermatology and aesthetic medicine. Since the development of the first dermaroller over 20 years ago, a variety of new microneedling devices have been introduced. Accordingly, the applications of microneedling in dermatology and aesthetic medicine have expanded indications over the past several years.

Evidence-based treatment of the skin for a variety of indications have been shown to be safe on all skin types. Microneedling is an effective modality of treatment, especially in patients with Fitzpatrick's IV and V skin types because it overcomes the side effects of scarring and hyperpigmentation resulting from other procedures in which the epidermis is compromised. It certainly promises to be a valuable technique with its numerous applications and its ever-expanding modifications.

References

1 Orentreich DS, Orentreich N. Subcutaneous incisionless (subcision) surgery for the correction of depressed scars and wrinkles. Dermatol Surg. 1995;21:543–549. [PubMed: 7773602]

2 Bahuguna A. Micro needling - Facts and Fictions. Asian J Med Sci. 2013;4:1–4.

3 Camirand A, Doucet J. Needle dermabrasion. Aesthet Plast Surg. 1997;21:48–51. [PubMed: 9204168]

4 Fernandes D. Minimally invasive percutaneous collagen induction. Oral Maxillofac Surg Clin North Am. 2006;17:51–63. [PubMed: 18088764]

5 Falabella AF, Falanga V.Wound healing. The Biology of the Skin. Parethenon: New York; 2001. pp. 281–299.

6 Fabbrocini G, Fardella N, Monfrecola A, et al. Acne scarring treatment using skin needling. Clinical and Experimental Dermatology. 2009;34:874–879.

7 Majid I, Sheikh G, September PI. Microneedling and its applications in dermatology InPrime. 7. Vol. 4. London: Informa Healthcare; 2014. Sep 15, pp. 44–49.

8 Aust MC, Fernandes D, Kolokythas P, et al. Percutaneous collagen induction therapy. An alternative treatment for scars, wrinkles, and skin laxity. Plast Reconstr Surg. 2008;121:1421–1429.

9 Nair PA, Arora TH. Microneedling using dermaroller: A means of collagen induction therapy. GMJ. 2014;69:24–27.

10 Jaffe L. Control of development by steady ionic currents. Fed Proc. 1981;40:125–127.

11 Aust MC, Reimers K, Gohritz A, et al. Percutaneous collagen induction. Scarless skin rejuvenation: fact or fiction? Clin Exp Dermatol. 2010 Jun;35(4):437–439.

12 Murata H, Zhou L, Ochoa S, et al. TGF-beta 3 stimulates and regulates collagen synthesis through TGF-beta-dependent and independent mechanisms. J Invest Dermatol. 1997;108:258–262.

13 Aust MC, Reimers K, Kaplan HM, et al. Percutaneous collagen induction regeneration in place of cicatrisation? J Plast Reconstr Aesthet Surg. 2011;64:97–107.

14 Zeitter S, Sikora Z, Jahn S, et al. Microneedling: Matching the results of medical needling and repetitive treatments to maximize potential for skin regeneration. Burns. 2014;40:966–973.

15 Aust MC, Knobloch K, Vogt PM. Percutaneous collagen induction as a novel therapeutic option for Striae distensae. Plast Reconstr Surg. 2010;126:4.

16 McCrudden MT, McAlister E, Courtenay AJ, et al. Microneedle applications in improving skin appearance. Exp Dermatol. 2015;24:561–566.

17 Arora S, Gupta BP. Automated microneedling device–A new tool in dermatologist's kit–A review. J Pak Med Assoc. 2012;22:354–357.

18 Doddaballapur S. Microneedling with dermaroller. J Cutan Aesthet Surg. 2009;2:110–111. [PMCID: PMC2918341] [PubMed: 20808602]

19 Anastassakis K. The Dermaroller Series. [Last accessed June 22, 2016] http://www.mtoimportadora.com.br/site_novo/wp.content/uploads/2014/04/Dr.-Anastassakis-Kostas.pdf.

20 Bhardwaj D. Collagen induction therapy with dermaroller. Community Based Med J. 2013;1:35–37.

21 McCrudden MT, McAlister E, Courtenay AJ, et al. Microneedle applications in improving skin appearance. Exp Dermatol. 2015;24:561–566. [PubMed: 25865925]

22 Lewis W. Is microneedling really the next big thing? Wendy Lewis explores the buzz surrounding skin needling. Plast Surg Pract. 2014;7:24–28.

2 A Short History of Skin Needling

Desmond Fernandes

Department of Plastic and Reconstructive Surgery, Faculty of Medicine, University of Cape Town

Introduction

I first started researching skin needling as we know it today in my medical practice in Cape Town on 20 volunteers starting in 1997. The treated cases had acne scarring, burn scars, and fine wrinkles. My first iteration of needling started in 1994 with deep dermal needling parallel to the skin surface of the upper lip skin to treat upper lip creases. This *horizontal* needling is not the same as subcision that Orentreich was doing for deep acne scars and wrinkles [1]. The two-year experience of this method was presented at the Asian Society of Aesthetic Plastic Surgery in Taipei in 1996.

Vertically oriented needling through the skin arose from the work of Camirand and Doucet for treating linear scars (e.g. face-lift scars) [2], which was discussed at the ISAPS meeting in São Paulo in 1997. I first started to use a tattoo artist's instrument, just as Camirand had (equivalent to the common pen-style needling done nowadays), to do needling of burn scars, wrinkles, and acne scars. That technique I found to be too laborious when doing the whole face and the needles could not penetrate as deeply as I felt they should. I also felt that the holes were too close to each other. That drove me to design a roller tool that I believed would be easier to use and give better, safer results.

I said the results of needling stemmed from the "inflammatory" cascade of growth factors and in particular TGF-beta-3 (TGFβ3), which had been described by Fergusson and his team as the regeneration factor [3]. I believed that a normal matrix was developed after needling to replace degenerated or scar collagen.

Microneedling: Global Perspectives in Aesthetic Medicine, First Edition.
Edited by Elizabeth Bahar Houshmand.
© 2021 John Wiley & Sons Ltd. Published 2021 by John Wiley & Sons Ltd.

My own personal histological studies had shown the increase of nonscar woven collagen and increased vertically oriented elastin. I also believed that vitamin A is so good for scars and regeneration of photoaged skin because of its stimulating growth factors [4–6].

Prof. Matthias Aust visited me in 2003, was intrigued by skin needling, and decided to research it at Hannover Medical School, Germany. His research subsequently revealed the platelet derived growth factors responsible for regeneration of the epidermis and matrix in rats in 2004 and was published in 2008 [7].

Today we know that skin needling is the safest way to treat scarred or aged skin and now we need to concentrate on the timing of needling and the chemicals we should use to promote better results. At this stage, vitamins A and C in the cosmetic form seems the best ingredients to use with needling, but research on the importance of selected peptides also offers great promise.

Because this chapter focuses on the history of skin needling, it necessarily includes a substantial autobiographical focus due to my role in bringing skin needling to the attention of the medical profession.

My clinical research in skin needing started in 1994 and at that time I was also trying to understand why cosmetic forms of vitamin A rejuvenated skin. I believed that growth factors had to be involved. However, I was also looking at the difficult problem of wrinkles/creases on the upper lip. I believed that these upper-lip lines were like scars between the skin and the deeper layer. I thought that if I could repeatedly pass a needle through the fibrous tissue under the lip lines and perforate them sufficiently they would then allow these "contractures" between the skin and the muscle to expand and thereby flatten out the wrinkles on the upper lip. That process was, in fact, the first iteration of skin needling, which I call *horizontal needling*. I still use this technique in conjunction with vertical needling.

I simply passed a needle backwards and forwards to create "tunnels" that were as close to the surface as I could manage and would thereby cause fenestration of any fibrous bands that were pulling in the wrinkles of the upper lip down to deeper tissue.

I started initially with a gauge 15 needle that I pierced through the upper-lip skin laterally and then pushed it medially backwards and forwards horizontally immediately under the skin. This is not the same as the subcision technique described by Orentreich, which completely transects scars or wrinkles away from the subcutaneous tissue [1]. I found that there were dense areas immediately under the wrinkles and I hoped the perforations into them would allow the skin to lift upwards. At that stage I thought we might make some scar tissue, but I did not think that we would cause tissue regeneration.

I did a presentation on my experience with skin needling with horizontal needling at the International Society of Plastic Surgery (ISAPS) meeting in 1996 in Taipei. I met Andre Camirand in São Paulo in 1997, when he mentioned that he could improve face-lift scars by "needle abrasion." He used a tattoo gun with a flat array of needles to abrade the scars that penetrated to the normal level used by tattoo artists. I then read his paper in which he spoke about piercing the skin vertically with a tattoo device to treat face-lift scars [2]. That made sense to me because until then I periodically struggled with hematomas that had formed under the skin, which meant that people were really uncomfortable because they had rather thick, bruised, lips that took time to settle. With vertical needling I had no problems like this.

I conducted the first research into skin needling as we know it today as part of my medical practice in Cape Town, working with 20 volunteers starting in 1997. My results convinced me to take skin needling into the realms of burn scars and photoaging wrinkles. The treated cases had acne scarring, burn scars, and fine wrinkles. Dr. Hilton Kaplan worked with me on virtually all of the early cases and we tried to explain why we were getting the results that we saw. I was impressed by the changes induced by skin needling and so were my patients, so it was easy to continue my research work and get more experience.

Since I was already looking at the question of why cosmetic versions of vitamin A rejuvenated skin, I came to the conclusion that both vitamin A and skin needling must be releasing growth factors. I was heavily influenced by the excellent research of Ferguson and his team, who were trying to prevent the formation of scars [3, 8]. His conclusion was that TGF-beta 3 (TGFβ3) was the dominant promoter of regeneration. His studies showed that TGF-beta 1 and 2 were the dominant growth factors in normal healing that causes scars. TGFβ3 makes only a transient appearance and disappears within 24 hours. In fetal wounds TGFβ3 dominates with Interleukin 10 (IL10) and hyaluronic acid, whereas TGFβ1 and TGFβ2 disappear rapidly. Ferguson felt that added TGFβ3 would change the paradigm of healing to scarless healing, i.e. regeneration. His results impressed me. In the case of skin needling the release of growth factors from platelets was much more intense than Vitamin A stimulating keratinocytes. However, at that stage we still had to wait for evidence that vitamin A stimulated growth factors, but eventually that was demonstrated [5]. Vitamin A is also one of the most powerful stimulants for hyaluronic acid production [9–11]. Since hyaluronic acid works synergistically with TGFβ3, this may be an important way that vitamin A helps improve scarring.

I first started to use a tattoo artist's instrument, just as Camirand had (equivalent to the common pen-style needling done nowadays) to do needling of burn scars, wrinkles, and acne scars. I recognized the risk of, but fortunately never experienced, excoriation of the epidermis because I had been professionally trained to do tattooing. I only wanted the needles to penetrate the blood vessels in the papillary dermis. That pen-type technique I found to be too laborious when doing the whole face and the needles could not penetrate as deeply as I felt they should. I also felt that the holes were too close together. I concluded that the needles needed to be longer so that they would prick not only the vessels of the upper papillary dermis but also those in the reticular dermis. For safety and to reduce skin resistance to penetration I needed needles more widely spaced apart in a roller-type device.

My aim was to get to the reticular dermis, which is about 1.0 mm below the surface of the skin on the face. That drove me in 1997 to design rollers with 1.0 to 3.0 mm length needles. I believe a roller tool is easier to use and gives better, safer results. I submitted the design for patent in 1998 but the idea could not be patented because Dr. Pistor (the "father" of mesotherapy) had designed and patented a very elegant stainless-steel roller with about 12 long sharp needles in the 1950s. I also designed a "patter" or stamper device, but I mainly used the rolling device.

My very first case of skin needling was to correct upper-lip creases. The patient was put onto vitamin A cosmetics and after three weeks I used regional anesthesia to numb her upper lip and I needled her upper lip intensively at 1.0 mm with the pen-style device. I covered the needled area with skin-colored micropore and asked her to apply the vitamin A cosmetics to the surface. She swelled considerably and after about five days I removed the micropore tapes and her lip looked intact but rather swollen. A month later I could see that the lip wrinkles looked better but not sufficiently so; therefore I advised a second needling done in the same way and after another month I felt that a third needling would give us a good result. By the end of the fourth month I was happy to sit back and wait for improvement. At that time, I realized that unlike laser treatments, where the results were obvious and best at about a month, with skin needling one needs to wait at least six months because there is progressive and well-defined improvement month after month. After that the changes are more subtle. In my first case, I was able to follow up for five years and I can say that if you do intensive needling together with applying vitamin A cosmetic skin care, then the excellent result can be maintained for at least four years, as shown in Figure 2.1.

While I started using a pen-type tattooing device, I felt that because the needle holes were too close together this produced a lot of inflammation. Once I started

(a)   (b)

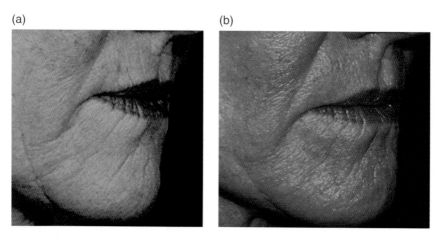

Figure 2.1 The very first case of needling; long-term result. (a) Before any treatment. (b) Four years after one needling per month for three sessions and continuous use of topical vitamin A and C. *Source:* Des Fernandes.

rolling I found that I got much less inflammation even after very intensive needling. After a few months I could see that the results were the same as those I got from using the pen-type of device. I found out that percutaneous needling is ideal to get changes in the reticular dermis and stimulate the production of collagen and elastin fibers.

Dr. Hugo Nel of Medunsa University was fascinated by the concept and did histology on roller-needled skin and reported to me personally that he could find no evidence of scar tissue and only found normal lattice-style collagen. Normal healthy dermal collagen is in a web or latticework and is not cross-linked, whereas scar collagen (cross-linked collagen III) is more densely laid down and the fibers lie in parallel bundles and are cross-linked. This was the first indication suggesting that skin needling caused regeneration instead of scarring. This was important evidence to support my concept that needling caused the release of platelet-derived growth factors (especially TGF-beta 3) and was responsible for regeneration as described by Ferguson.

My classical technique of skin needling using a roller

The roller is the safest and most effective way to needle the whole face, stretch marks, deep acne scars, or burn scars. I generally don't use it for linear scars or fresh scars, where I prefer to use the pen-style device. I also use the pen-style device when I needle the upper eyelids and close to the lower eyelid's eyelashes. I believe we should all become expert in using both techniques. The roller device is far easier to use and requires less training.

By rolling backwards and forwards in various directions, or by repeatedly rolling in one direction with some pressure, one can achieve an even distribution of holes. The skin should be kept taught and be needled as densely as possible to maximize the release of platelets and hence the secretion of growth factors. Usually, as the needle holes get too close to each other, the needle "slips" into an established hole and so it seems impossible to overtreat the skin and make the holes too close to each other. The needles penetrate right through the epidermis but do not excoriate or remove it, so the epidermis is only punctured and will rapidly heal. Histological studies show that the needle seems mainly to divide cells from each other rather than cutting through the cells, so many cells are spared injury. The epidermis and particularly the stratum corneum remain intact, except for these tiny holes, which are about four cells in diameter. The needles penetrate about 1.5 to 2 mm into the dermis. Naturally, the skin bleeds for a short time, but that soon stops.

Contrary to popular myth, the needle holes are simple, and the skin never gets slits or cuts as the needle exits the skin. I have examined this very carefully and studied it with slow motion video. The skin is tented upwards as the needle lifts the skin but then because the roller is moving in the opposite direction the needle simply slides out of the skin. There is only one hole through which the blood may escape, and I believe more blood (and platelets) remain in the skin and hence could give a better final result. The more platelets, the richer the concentration of platelet-derived growth factors. The skin develops multiple microbruises in the dermis that initiate the complex cascade of growth factors that results in collagen production. One advantage of the roller that can never be replicated by the mechanical pen-type devices is that through one hole many arterioles are cut or pierced as the needle transits from entrance to exit. This is very different from when one uses a vertical stamper or pen device: each punctured blood vessel is under a hole through which blood may escape and potentially less blood remains in the dermis. The mechanical devices merely penetrate the blood vessels immediately in the vertical pathway of the needle.

After the bleeding stops, there is a serous ooze that must to be wiped from the surface of the skin. Wet gauze swabs soak up most of this serous ooze. As the skin swells, the holes are closed, the edges of the epidermis are approximated, and the ooze stops. Chemicals, however, may still penetrate the skin, so only safe molecules should be used topically. After this serous leak has stopped, the skin is washed and then covered with vitamins A and C [12]. There is no other special postneedling care, but I have found that exposing the skin to a low pH immediately after needling seems to facilitate even better results.

When I had sufficient histology to prove in my own clinical cases that we were regenerating skin, I understood that – for the first time in medical history – a medical intervention could cause regeneration instead of scar formation when treating scars or photodamaged skin. Till then all other treatments, such as CO2 laser or heavy peeling, had focused on scarring skin to tighten and smoothen it. In fact, skin needling is also known as percutaneous collagen induction (PCI)_ therapy and the automatic production particularly of TGF-beta 3 opened up a new paradigm in treating scars.

I collected enough evidence to present a paper at the International Confederation for Plastic, Reconstructive & Aesthetic Surgery (IPRAS) meeting in San Francisco in June 1999 and the presentation was acclaimed by the packed audience as a breakthrough in treating scarring. Although I had pointed out that all my cases were prepared for a minimum of three months with a topical cosmetic vitamin A equivalent to retinoic acid 0.025 to 0.05 g%, few people recognized the value of preparation of the skin and so several months later I had complaints from several doctors who said needling did not make impressive changes. On questioning about what skin care they used, they generally said, "Come on, we all know that cosmetics do not work." The other point that they missed was that needling has to be done quite intensively to make real changes.

I lectured around the world at international plastic surgery and aesthetic meetings and was invited to publish the first paper on skin needling as an alternative to laser treatments of skin in the Aesthetic Surgery Journal in 2002 [13]. At one meeting in Tokyo, Andre Camirand was told about my concept of growth factors causing the changes and after giving it thought for a minute he confessed that he had missed that detail, but of course he was looking at small areas and thought that needling restored normal skin color by transplanting melanocytes that adhered to the needle.

Prof. Matthias Aust, who visited me in 2003, was intrigued by skin needling and he decided to research it at Hannover Medical School, Germany. He confirmed in 2004 that platelet-derived growth factors cause regeneration in rats (his work was finally published in 2010) [14]. We also published our combined experience of the clinical results in over 480 humans to show that needling was a valid way to treat wrinkles, stretch marks, and scars [15]. Aust continued his exploration of needling for various conditions [7, 16–23]. He particularly concentrated on burn scars and was awarded the European Burn Society Gold Medal for his work in treating burn scars. The lesson I learned from Aust was that because TGFβ3 is raised for only two weeks, even better results could be achieved by reducing the intervals between needling and so I slowly started to change the frequency of treatments until I felt safe doing 1.0 mm needling once a week. I tried 0.5 mm needling without topical anesthesia and that did not cause enough bleeding into the papillary dermis. If I did an intensive 0.5 mm needling with topical anesthesia I could manage to cause enough bleeding but I preferred needles at 0.8, 0.9, and 1.0 mm because I could get good bleeding without discomfort for the patient. I found that topical anesthetics, e.g. EMLA, made 1.0 mm needling very acceptable. I discovered that one has to make certain adjustments to enable topical anesthetic to work better. All topical anesthetics are kept in an acidic base to preserve activity. However, anesthetics function well only at an alkaline pH. For that reason, I devised a technique using a product I formulated to make the skin surface more alkaline before applying the topical anesthetic product. As a result, one gets much more intense anesthesia that may even allow 3.0 mm needling.

I realized that I could only do once-a-week needling with a roller because when I tried to do it with a pen-type device the swelling and inflammation were too marked for the patients to tolerate that regimen. Needling, on the other hand, done under topical anesthesia, generally allowed the patients to return to work the day after the treatment.

At the invitation of Dr. Joe Niamtu, who heard me lecture on skin needling in Australia, I published my second article on minimally invasive collagen induction [24]. Dr. Massimo Signorini in Milan, Italy, was one of the first to understand the efficacy of skin needling in treating photoaging and started collecting his results from skin needling. Soon after that, we were able to publish an article together [12]. Hilton Kaplan, who had worked with me on many of my earlier cases, was eventually able, with Dr. Julie Kenner from California, to present our combined multicenter work at the American Academy of Dermatology in 2006. When my results started to gain attention the roller design was adopted by many companies around the world.

In the beginning of my work with microneedling I said that the induction of the inflammatory phase following wounding was the best way to describe the concatenation of chemical events following the release of platelets and the platelet-derived growth factors. Today I regret using that word because needling does not cause significant inflammation, yet several "experts" say that the frequent needling sessions that I advise "overwhelm" the skin system because of excessive inflammation and that interferes with the final results. I have pointed out repeatedly that I, and my patients, do not see the degree of inflammation that we encountered when I did pen-type needling, and the results I achieved with more frequent needling set the standard for what could be achieved by skin needling. Some of my patients have demanded less frequent treatments than what I consider ideal, and so I have also built up a comparative experience and can say without prejudice that six needlings done at one-month intervals gives an inferior result compared to doing six needlings spread over five weeks (5–6-day intervals). Needling causes a healing cascade of growth factors totally unrelated to the inflammation caused by prostaglandins and inflammazones and is totally driven by the platelet-derived growth factors.

My research has been a continuous voyage from 1998 till the present. Today I believe the roller is the safest way to treat thicker scars. Lasers, etc. do not give competitive results. Pen-style needling cannot penetrate the skin and scar tissue properly and may cause damage to the epidermis in trying to do this depth of needling.

I have tried to find out:

1 what length needles were required for various scars, wrinkles and stretchmarks,
2 which chemicals were the best for using before and after needling,
3 the best time intervals in between needling sessions, and
4 how we can use skin needling immediately after surgery to help make almost invisible scars.

We need to investigate when and how to needle an incision. Either before the elected surgery (one week before, one day before, or even immediately before the incision is made) or after surgery. This could be immediately after the wound has been sutured closed, or when sutures/dressings are removed.

Another use for needling could be acute burn injuries. The growth factors released could speed up the regeneration of the tissue and could also help to improve immune defense. Maybe scar contractures could be avoided. The possibility of using needling in skin graft donor sites may offer the chance of less visible scars and even the opportunity to reharvest skin from the same donor area.

The appearance of cellulite has also been treated successfully with needling. The PCI effectively tightens up the skin again and smoothens the surface.

The best chemicals to be used

Vitamin A

Because I have clinically researched vitamin A since 1982, and I knew that cosmetic vitamin A changes scars and seems to make normal-looking skin, it was sensible for me to prepare all my cases for needling by asking them to apply progressively stronger concentrations of vitamin A. By about three months the patients were using retinyl palmitate with concentrations in international units equivalent to retinoic acid 0.025 g% at the minimum but going up even to retinoic acid 0.1 g%. I purposely formulated the vitamin A creams in international units to ensure good DNA activity. I also believed that we were relying on the fibroblasts to make the changes so it made sense to "supercharge" the fibroblasts and make them ready for the intense activity that would follow needling. I believe the results I achieved validated the necessity to use vitamin A before and after skin needling. We know vitamin A also hastens healing, normalizes skin cells, and promotes normal collagen in a lattice pattern [5, 25–30].

Vitamin C

Vitamin C is essential for the production of normal collagen and even activates genes related to collagen production [31–35], and since we were stimulating the system to produce more collagen, that automatically means that one needs more vitamin C [36, 37]. I have generally used ascorbyl-tetraisopalmitate in my formulations because it is to date the most effective way of getting vitamin C into fibroblasts [38–40].

Selected peptides

Cosmetic peptides have in recent years become very effective – ever since the introduction of the pioneering Matrixyl abut 20 years ago. I believe effective cocktails of newer peptides will offer even greater chances for better results (see Figure 2.2).

The frequency of needling

The most convincing research on the frequency of needling comes from Aust's research at Hannover Medical School. Of particular note for addressing this controversial topic is the report by Zeitter [41]. The researchers were able to compare the results of 3 mm needling done once a month for a total of for four sessions with 1 mm needling done once a week for a total of four sessions. The weekly needling gave superior results. They also showed conclusively that vitamins A and C gave up to almost four times better thickening of the skin.

(a)   (b)

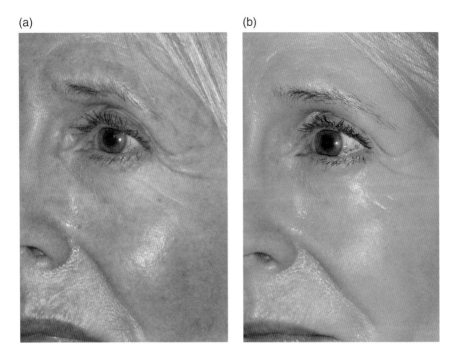

Figure 2.2 Long-term effects of skin needling with a 1.0 mm roller and using vitamins A and C and selected peptides. (a) Before: At 67 years of age the patient had a series of six needlings done in five weeks and concomitantly had facials to infuse vitamins A and C and peptides by using iontophoresis and low-frequency sonophoresis. (b) After: Four years after completing the treatment and maintaining her skincare, one can see the skin has been lifted, and is smoother and more youthful looking. Pigment marks have also faded. *Source:* Des Fernandes.

Conclusion

In the beginning doctors dismissed skin needling as a simple, ineffective medieval torture but, fortunately, through continuous research, skin needling has become a valuable, inexpensive tool that can be used around the world in the most primitive conditions for the most important rehabilitative work, or for rejuvenation. It will probably remain a valuable tool for many years in the future.

References

1 Orentreich DS, Orentreich N. Subcutaneous incisionless (subcision) surgery for the correction of depressed scars and wrinkles. Dermatol Surg. 1995;21(6):543–549.
2 Camirand A, Doucet J. Needle dermabrasion. Aesthetic Plast Surg. 1997;21(1):48–51.
3 O'Kane S, Ferguson MW. Transforming growth factor beta s and wound healing. Int J Biochem Cell Biol. 1997;29(1):63–78.

4 Polcz ME, Barbul A. The Role of Vitamin A in Wound Healing. Nutr Clin Pract. 2019;34(5):695–700.

5 Shao Y, He T, Fisher GJ, et al. Molecular basis of retinol anti-ageing properties in naturally aged human skin in vivo. Int J Cosmet Sci, 2017. 39(1):56–65.

6 Kafi R, Kwak HSR, Schumacher WE, et al. Improvement of naturally aged skin with vitamin A (retinol). Arch Dermatol. 2007;143(5):606–612.

7 Aust MC, Fernandes D, Kolokythas P, et al. Percutaneous collagen induction therapy: an alternative treatment for scars, wrinkles, and skin laxity. Plast Reconstr Surg. 2008;121(4):1421–1429.

8 Shah M, Foreman DM, Ferguson MW. Neutralisation of TGF-beta 1 and TGF-beta 2 or exogenous addition of TGF-beta 3 to cutaneous rat wounds reduces scarring. Journal of Cell Science. 1995;10(Pt 3):985–1002.

9 Saavalainen K, Pasonen-Seppänen S, Dunlop TW, et al. The human hyaluronan synthase 2 gene is a primary retinoic acid and epidermal growth factor responding gene. J Biol Chem. 2005;280(15):14636–14644.

10 Chen S, Beehler B, Sugimoto G, Tramposch KM. Effects of all-trans retinoic acid on glycosaminoglycan synthesis in photodamaged hairless mouse skin. J Invest Dermatol. 1993;101(2):237–239.

11 King IA. Increased epidermal hyaluronic acid synthesis caused by four retinoids. Br J Dermatol. 1984;110(5):607–608.

12 Fernandes D, Signorini M. Combating photoaging with percutaneous collagen induction. Clin Dermatol. 2008;26(2):192–199.

13 Fernandes D. Percutaneous collagen induction: an alternative to laser resurfacing. Aesthet Surg J. 2002;22(3):307–309.

14 Aust MC, Reimers K, Gohritz A, et al. Percutaneous collagen induction. Scarless skin rejuvenation: fact or fiction? Clin Exp Dermitol. 2010;35(4):437–439.

15 European Academy of Dermatology and Venereology Congress. Photodamaged skin: clinical management with topical tretinoin. Proceedings of a satellite symposium to the 1st congress of the European Academy of Dermatology and Venereology. Florence, 26 September 1989. in J Int Med Res. 1990.

16 Aust MC, Reimers K, Repenning C, et al. Percutaneous collagen induction: minimally invasive skin rejuvenation without risk of hyperpigmentation - fact or fiction? Plast Reconstr Surg. 2008;122(5):1553–1563.

17 Aust MC, Reimers K, Vogt PM. Medical needling: improving the appearance of hypertrophic burn scars. GMS Verbrennungsmedizin. 2009;3:Doc 03.

18 Aust MC, Knobloch K, Gohritz A, et al. Percutaneous collagen induction therapy for hand rejuvenation. Plast Reconstr Surg. 2010;126(4):203e-204e.

19 Aust MC, Knobloch K, Vogt PM. Percutaneous collagen induction therapy as a novel therapeutic option for Striae distensae. Plast Reconstr Surg. 2010;126(4):219e-220e.

20 Aust MC, Reimers K, Kaplan HM, et al. Percutaneous collagen induction-regeneration in place of cicatrisation? J Plast Reconstr Aesthet Surg. 2010.

21 Aust MC, Reimers K, Kaplan HM, et al. Percutaneous collagen induction-regeneration in place of cicatrisation? J Plast Reconstr Aesthet Surg. 2011;64(1):97–107.

22 Aust MC, Bathe S, Fernandes D. Illustrated guide to percutaneous collagen induction: Basics, Indications, Uses. 2013. United Kingdom: Quintessence Publishing.

23 Aust MC, Walezko N. Acne scars and striae distensae: Effective treatment with medical skin needling. Hautarzt. 2015;66(10):748–752.

24 Fernandes D. Minimally invasive percutaneous collagen induction. Oral Maxillofac Surg Clin North Am. 2005;17(1):51–63.

25 Kang S. The mechanism of action of topical retinoids. Cutis. 2005;75(2 Suppl):10–3; discussion 13.

26 Sorg O, Kuenzli S, Kaya G, Saurat JH. Proposed mechanisms of action for retinoid derivatives in the treatment of skin aging. J Cosmet Dermatol. 2005;4(4):237–244.

27 Griffiths CE. The role of retinoids in the prevention and repair of aged and photoaged skin. Clin Exp Dermatol. 2001;26(7): 613–618.

28 Sorg O, Antille C, Kaya G, Saurat JH. Retinoids in cosmeceuticals. Dermatol Ther. 2006;19(5):289–296.

29 Antille C, Tran C, Sorg O, Saurat JH. Penetration and metabolism of topical retinoids in ex vivo organ-cultured full-thickness human skin explants. Skin Pharmacol Physiol. 2004;17(3):124–128.

30 Antille C, Tran C, Sorg O, et al. Vitamin A exerts a photoprotective action in skin by absorbing ultraviolet B radiation. J Invest Dermatol. 2003;121(5):1163–1167.

31 Pinnell SR, Murad S, Darr D. Induction of collagen synthesis by ascorbic acid. A possible mechanism. Arch Dermatol. 1987;123(12):1684–1686.

32 Geesin JC, Darr D, Kaufman R, et al. Ascorbic acid specifically increases type I and type III procollagen messenger RNA levels in human skin fibroblast. J Invest Dermatol. 1988;90(4):420–424.

33 Geesin JC, Hendricks LJ, Gordon JS, Berg RA. Modulation of collagen synthesis by growth factors: the role of ascorbate-stimulated lipid peroxidation. Arch Biochem Biophys. 1991;289(1):6–11.

34 Nusgens BV, Humbert P, Rougier A, et al. Topically applied vitamin C enhances the mRNA level of collagens I and III, their processing enzymes and tissue inhibitor of matrix metalloproteinase 1 in the human dermis. J Invest Dermatol. 2001;116(6):853–859.

35 Duarte TL, Cooke MS, Jones G. Gene expression profiling reveals new protective roles for vitamin C in human skin cells. Free Radic Biol Med. 2009;46(1):78–87.

36 Tajima S, Pinnell SR. Ascorbic acid preferentially enhances type I and III collagen gene transcription in human skin fibroblasts. J Dermatol Sci. 1996;11(3):250–253.

37 Moores J. Vitamin C: a wound healing perspective. Br J Community Nurs, 2013;Suppl:S6, S8–11.

38 Machado NCF, Dos Santos L, Carvalho BG, et al. Assessment of penetration of Ascorbyl Tetraisopalmitate into biological membranes by molecular dynamics. Comput Biol Med. 2016;75:151–159.

39 Campos PM, Goncalves GM, Gaspar LR. In vitro antioxidant activity and in vivo efficacy of topical formulations containing vitamin C and its derivatives studied by non-invasive methods. Skin Res Technol. 2008;14(3):376–380.

40 Gaspar LR, Maia Campos PMBG. Photostability and efficacy studies of topical formulations containing UV-filters combination and vitamins A, C and E International Journal of Pharmaceutics. 343(1–2).

41 Zeitter S, Sikora Z, Jahn S, et al. Microneedling: Matching the results of medical needling and repetitive treatments to maximize potential for skin regeneration. Burns: Journal of the International Society for Burn Injuries. 2014;40(5):966–973.

3 The Value of Medical Needling in Burn Scars

Matthias Aust[1], Desmond Fernandes[2], and Richard Bender[3]

[1] Aust Aesthetik, Landsberg am Lech, Germany
[2] Department of Plastic and Reconstructive Surgery, Faculty of Medicine, University of Cape Town
[3] St. Vinzenz Hospital, Cologne, Germany

Introduction

Patients with burn scar deformities frequently request help to improve both the aesthetic and functional complications of their scars. There are numerous methods available for surgeons to treat burn scars, but nowadays there is a demand for less invasive and more cost-effective procedures to give the desired benefits.

Noninvasive treatments such as silicone patches and pressure garments are important ways to control scars. Minimally invasive techniques such as cortisone injections also have a place. Surgeons have generally depended on surgical interventions such as scar excision, W- or Z-plasties, and pedicled or free skin flaps to treat contractures or severe irregular scars. The quest for better results has also led to the application of many different topical therapies, such as laser resurfacing, dermabrasion, and deep chemical peels.

The aforementioned methods all follow the same principal: they are ablative; they change the scar by destroying the epidermis partially or completely and scarring the dermis. The death of tissue leads to an inflammatory response. In the process of trying to treat dermal scarring the epidermis may be completely destroyed and replaced by a thinner epidermis with flatter rete ridges covering parallel-oriented scar collagen, which is distinctive for scarred skin [1–3]. Furthermore, the skin becomes more vulnerable to infections [4].

The ideal scar-treatment method would avoid ablation of the epidermis, and rather promote the formation of physiological dermal collagen in a lattice pattern by initiating the expression of growth factors which are relevant for scarless wound healing and regeneration of the skin. In other words, the perfect remedy would be to remove the visible defective scarring and regenerate healthier, anatomically more normal skin.

Microneedling: Global Perspectives in Aesthetic Medicine, First Edition.
Edited by Elizabeth Bahar Houshmand.
© 2021 John Wiley & Sons Ltd. Published 2021 by John Wiley & Sons Ltd.

In recent years it has been proven possible, to a significant degree, to achieve the ideal treatment by using percutaneous collagen induction or "medical needling" [5–7]. Medical needling is a minimally invasive nonablative procedure capable of improving scar quality and functionality by dermal reorganization, with a decrease in scar collagen accompanied by an increase of physiological collagen and fibronectin as well as an increase of glycosaminoglycans. There is a decrease of transepidermal water loss because the epidermis is thicker and the stratum corneum becomes a fully functional water barrier.

Approximately 20 years ago Camirand and Doucet demonstrated that by simple "needle abrasion" one could get significant clinical improvement in treating white surgical scars with a tattoo artist's device [8]. Orentreich also reported on "dermal needling or subcision" as an alternative for treating scars and wrinkles [9]. Based on these concepts, Fernandes developed the percutaneous collagen induction technique [10]. Thanks to targeted research within the last 15 years, impressive scientific data is now available which underlines the efficacy and safety of medical needling and why it works [5, 7, 11–15].

Science

How it works

Medical needling is repetitive puncturing of burn scars with a roller equipped with 3.0 mm-long needles that penetrate into the dermal scars and cause intradermal bleeding (see Figure 3.1).

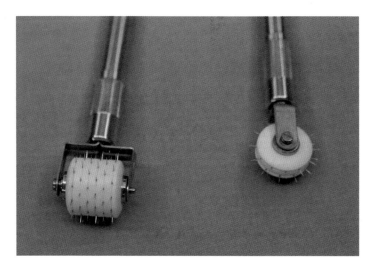

Figure 3.1 Needling device. *Source:* Matthias Aust.

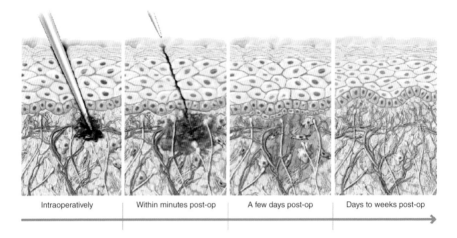

| Intraoperatively | Within minutes post-op | A few days post-op | Days to weeks post-op |

Figure 3.2 Schematic illustration of medical needling and the effects on the wound. The needle pierces the epidermis and the blood vessels of the dermis. When the needle is withdrawn the needle tract closes and by the next day it cannot be detected histologically. Within days collagen I and elastin are generated.

The needling device is repeatedly rolled over the scar in three main directions – longitudinally, diagonally, and horizontally – to get the best distribution of puncture holes. According to the extent of the scar, this procedure can last 30 minutes or longer. It is important to use the device with constant pressure and to do the rolling in one direction at a time to prevent shear forces. The needles are solid and do not have a lumen. Hence, they pierce the skin and mainly separate the skin cells rather than destroying them (see Figure 3.2). They penetrate the dermis 2–3 mm and produce thousands of micropuncture wounds and intradermal bleeding. Some blood comes up through the channels to cause bleeding on the surface. The most important bleeding occurs in the dermis but bleeding through the skin gives us a good idea of what is happening below in the dermis.

Induction of the wound-healing cascade

This trauma initiates the activation of the physiological wound-healing cascade but with a significant difference form the norm. Normally trauma causes the temporary presence of TGFβ3 and the wound heals predominantly under the influence of TGFβ1 and -β2, which results in scar tissue. After needling TGFβ-1 and -β-2 rapidly disappear from the scene and TGFβ3 dominates, resulting in scarless healing and regeneration [16]. Skin needling induces a new (and as yet unrecognized) phase of regenerative healing which should not be confused with the post-traumatic inflammatory cascade. Platelets, keratinocytes, and neutrophils secrete growth factors such as platelet-derived growth factor (PDGF), fibroblast growth factor (FGF), vascular endothelial growth factor (VEGF), tissue growth factor, and transforming growth factor-α and -ß (TGFα, TGFß). These initiate the synthesis of dermal structures such as collagen, elastin, and fibronectin and stimulate the migration of fibroblasts and keratinocytes 13 [17]. The modulation of these growth factors right at the beginning signal the differences between this new paradigm of scarless healing and the archetypal healing with scar formation.

TGF and the induction of collagen I

This new repair and regeneration mechanism is relevant for the formation of collagen I, which is the physiological-type collagen in a lattice pattern in healthy skin, whereas collagen III is more prevalent in parallel-oriented scar collagen. TGFβ3 makes a transient presence in standard surgical wounds and has largely disappeared within 24 hours of injury. Typical scars, we now know, are the result of dominant activity of TGFß1 and -2. In contrast, TGFß1 and -2 levels are extremely low in scarless embryonal wound healing while the levels of TGFß3 are remarkably high [1, 5, 16, 18].

Medical needling particularly influences the liberation of TGFß1, -2, and -3. Within days post-treatment the levels of TGFß1 and -2 are significantly downregulated whereas TGFß3 reaches high expression levels even beyond the initial wound-healing phase [7, 13]. In support of this, the production of type I collagen was found to be increased after medical needling (see Figures 3.3–3.5). The changes seen with skin needling indicate a lower level of TGFß3 by two months. Ferguson's team argues that the initial height of the rise in TGFß3 concentration is probably the most important influence, not so much the duration of the raised levels because the TGFß3 does not stay raised for the extended healing period [19]. Studies in humans that are as yet unpublished show that TGFß3 is raised after needling and become higher when needling is done at short intervals (Fernandes, personal communication).

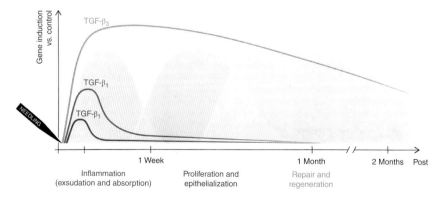

Figure 3.3 Microarray analyses of TGFß1, -2, and -3 expression levels in treated animals. The induction of TGFß3 gene expression continues even beyond the initial wound-healing phase, whereas TGFß1 and -2 are downregulated during the second week post-treatment.

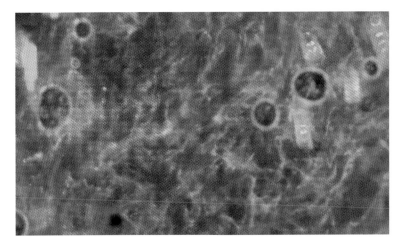

Figure 3.4 Immunofluorescence visualization of collagen I: Staining with antibodies directed against Collagen I (Alexa488) and DAPI. Un-needled animal of the dermis failed to react with the antibodies. *Source:* Matthias Aust.

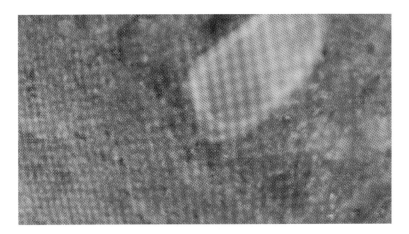

Figure 3.5 Immunhistochemical staining, anti–collagen I. Needled animal with eight weeks of skincare stained without primary antibody. The amount of type I collagen was qualitatively increased in the treated group compared to their controls, judged by the brighter fluorescence. *Source:* Matthias Aust.

Dermal remodeling

Dermal reorganization after medical needling depends not only on the formation of physiological oriented collagen I but also on the inclusion of glycosaminogly-can molecules and fibronectin. This was shown in the animal model through the quantitative analysis of gene expression as well as through immunohistological analyses [13, 20, 21]. As seen in Figures 3.12 and 3.13, the entire connective tissue framework appears thicker and denser post-treatment.

Increase in skin elasticity

Moreover, the stimulation of the endogenous FGF contributes to improved skin elasticity. As seen in Figures 3.6 and 3.7, the amount of elastin is significantly higher after medical needling.

Normalized perfusion

The secretion of VEGF during the healing phase stimulates angiogenesis and leads to the formation of tiny blood vessels in the corium. This helps to normalize the characteristic pathological erythema of scars after burn injuries. As seen in Figures 3.8 and 3.9, the amount of VEGF significantly rises after medical needling.

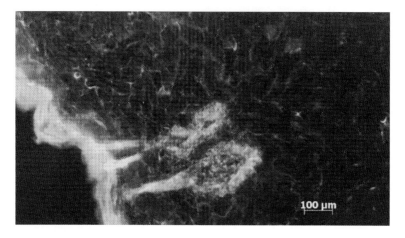

Figure 3.6 Immunhistochemical staining, antielastin. Untreated animal immunofluorescence visualization of elastin: Staining with antibodies directed against elastin (Alexa488) and DAPI. Un-needled animal of the dermis failed to react with the antibodies. *Source:* Matthias Aust.

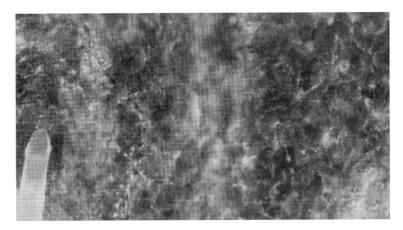

Figure 3.7 Immunhistochemical staining, antielastin. Needled animal with eight weeks of skincare stained without primary antibody. The amount of elastin was qualitatively increased in the treated group compared to their controls, judged by the brighter fluorescence. *Source:* Matthias Aust.

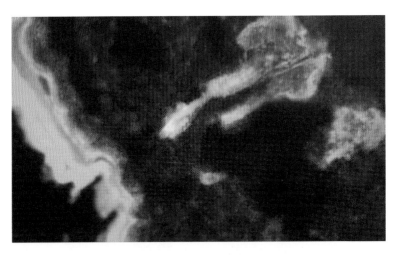

Figure 3.8 Immunhistochemical staining, anti-VEGF. Untreated animal immunofluorescence visualization of elastin: Staining with antibodies directed against elastin (Alexa488) and DAPI. Un-needled animal of the dermis failed to react with the antibodies. *Source:* Matthias Aust.

Increase in skin moisture content

Scars often appear dry and loose due to a decrease of glycosaminoglycans with a result of reduced water retention in the skin and due to thinner epidermis with increased transepidermal water loss. Medical needling is associated with a higher inclusion of glycosaminoglycans (see Figures 3.10 and 3.11) and with a thicker epidermis post-treatment (see Figures 3.12 and 3.13). Both help to maximize the moisture of the skin back to the reference of healthy skin.

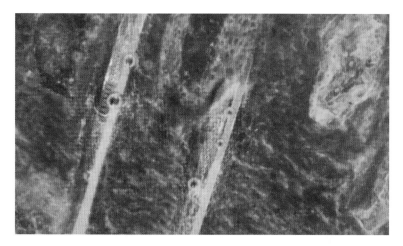

Figure 3.9 Immunhistochemical staining, anti-VEGF. Needled animal. VEGF showed a membranous staining pattern along the intercellular junctions in the basal and suprabasal layers of the epidermis. A brighter fluorescence indicates that the amount of VEGF in the dermis is augmented in the needled groups compared to the un-needled groups. *Source:* Matthias Aust.

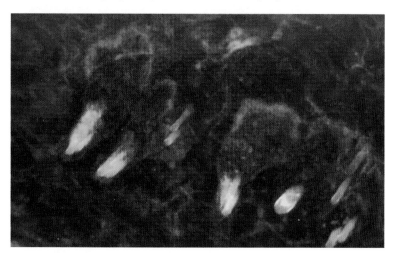

Figure 3.10 Immunofluorescence visualization of GAGs (Alexa488-conjugated) and DAPI (representative example). Un-needled animal with eight weeks of skincare. GAGs showed dense deposits occupying much of the dermis, leaving only isolated collagen bundles visible. *Source:* Matthias Aust.

Increase of epidermal thickness

In contrast to ablative treatments, the skin structures are not injured after medical needling. The epidermis remains physiologically intact, which means that potential side effects such as inflammation, new scarring, or dyspigmentation are reduced to a minimum. Furthermore, it has been shown in the animal model that the thickness of the epidermis increases up to 140% after treatment versus untreated ones [22]. (See Figures 3.12 and 3.13.)

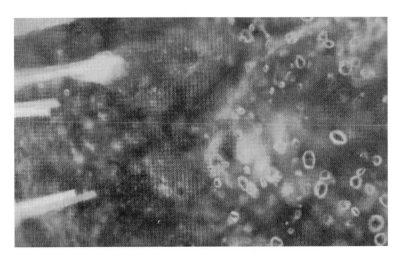

Figure 3.11 Immunhistochemical staining, anti-GAG. Needled animal with eight weeks of skincare stained without primary antibody. As observed in the PAS staining, a marked increase in the amount of GAGs was observed throughout the different needled groups in comparison to the un-needled groups. *Source:* Matthias Aust.

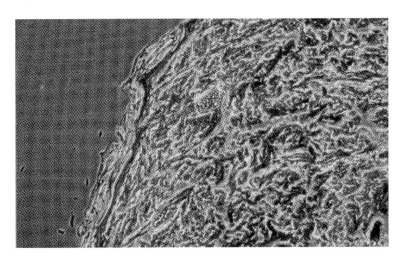

Figure 3.12 Masson's trichrome staining. Untreated animal (control). *Source:* Matthias Aust.

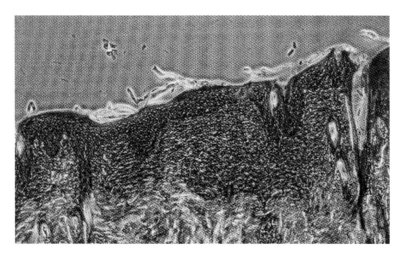

Figure 3.13 Needled animal with eight weeks of skincare. Collagen fiber bundles were increased, thickened, and more loosely woven in both the papillary and reticular dermis, most prominently in the needled plus skincare group. Elastin fibers in the dermis were highly linear and the epidermal dermal interface showed regular dermal papillae; cellular polarity and normal epidermal differentiation appeared to be maintained; and the elastin network within the reticular dermis was regularly thickened and organized in all groups. *Source:* Matthias Aust.

Role of vitamins in wound healing

Maximal post-needling improvement was seen in combination with pre- and post-treatment of the skin with vitamin A and oxidants Vitamin C and E (see Figures 3.12 and 3.13).

No dyspigmentation after medical needling

A disadvantage of ablative scar treatments is that there is an increased risk of dyspigmentation, especially in darker skin types [23–25]. On 480 patients, it has been shown that there is no risk of dyspigmentation after medical needling [26]. Furthermore, medical needling does not change the number of melano-cytes but the expression levels of melanocyte-stimulating hormone (MSH) and Interleukin-10 (Il-10) are modified [26]. MSH, which influences the prolifera-tion and activity of melanocytes, is significantly downregulated within days after treatment. Il-10 as an anti-inflammatory cytokine is upregulated postoperatively [20]. In a subsequent study, it has been shown that it is not possible to repigment larger areas of hypopigmented skin with medical needling alone.

Repigmentation of hypopigmented burn scars with medical needling and non-cultured autologous skin cell suspension (NCASCS)

Currently numerous methods are available to treat hypopigmented skin, such as split skin grafting [27, 28], lasers [29], and cultured skin cell transplantation [30–32]. In recent years, research focused additionally on noncultured skin cell suspension. The autologous cell harvesting device is used to create a spray suspension of living autologous skin cells. These cells are harvested intraoperatively and directly applied, in suspension, to the prepared wound.

In order to prepare an area for treatment with NCASCS, the wound has been first treated by using dermabrasion or lasers, which are both ablative methods. By their nature, ablative treatments remove skin structures and cells, including the basement membrane, which are replaced by a thinner epidermis with flatter rete ridges [1, 2, 32]. This initiates an inflammatory response that stimulates fibroblasts to produce parallel oriented scar collagen instead of physiological lattice-pattern collagen [1, 33]. Additionally, the risk of dyspigmentation increases after these ablative treatments due to associated damage to the melanocytes [34, 35].

An ideal wound preparation for the autologous cell suspension would be a treatment that does not destroy structures of the epidermis yet creates a conduit that allows ingress of melanocytes, but that promotes the formation of physiological collagen instead of scar collagen and initiates the expression of growth factors. As described above, medical needling offers all these advantages.

To combine both procedures it is at first necessary to prepare a depigmented scar with intense medical needling. Afterwards the autologous cell suspension is applied through a spray syringe on the wound.

The hypothesis is that the melanocytes of the cell suspension link through the epidermal canals onto the basal membrane. In a pilot study with 20 patients it has been shown that it is possible to get marked subjective and objective improvements regarding repigmentation with the combination of medical needling and NCASCS [36].

Clinical results

The following images show the clinical results of microneedling therapy for a variety of skin conditions.

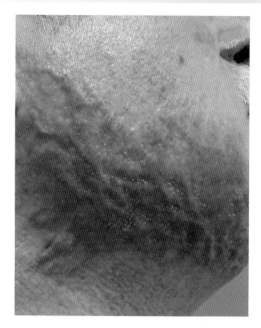

Figure 3.14 One-month-old active burn scar due to open fire burn injury. Note the active, hypertrophic, stiff and red scarring. *Source:* Matthias Aust

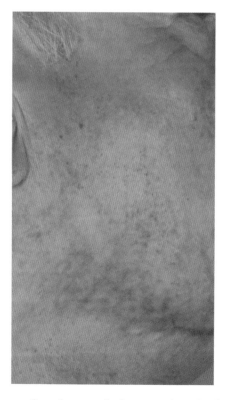

Figure 3.15 Needling was performed one month after trauma (just after the epithelium was closed). Picture shows improvement of the scar one year post-needling. *Source:* Matthias Aust

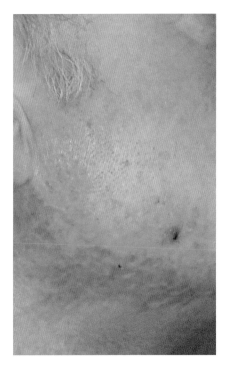

Figure 3.16 Result after a second deep needling one year after the second needling (two years post–initial trauma). *Source:* Matthias Aust.

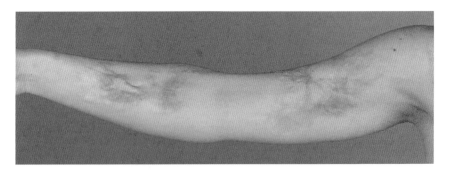

Figure 3.17 Hypertrophic burn scar, lower arm, 5 years post-trauma. *Source:* Matthias Aust.

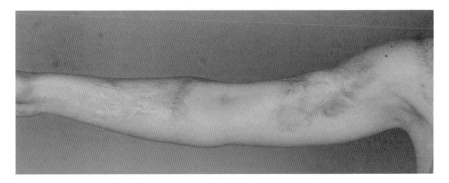

Figure 3.18 Improvement of the hypertrophic burn scar six months post–3mm needling. *Source:* Matthias Aust.

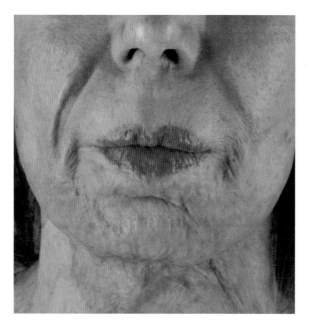

Figure 3.19 Full Face burn scars after a deep second- and third-degree burn accident. Picture taken 10 years post-trauma. *Source:* Matthias Aust.

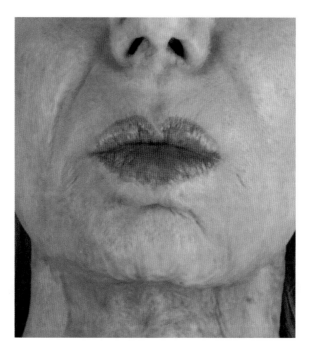

Figure 3.20 Improvement of the skin and scar condition six months after a 3mm needling of the face. *Source:* Matthias Aust.

Medical needling and ncascs

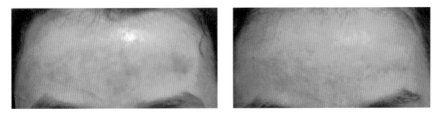

Figure 3.21 Forehead scar with hypopigmented areas before and with better repigmentation one year post-needling combined with NCASCS. *Source:* Matthias Aust.

(a)   (b)

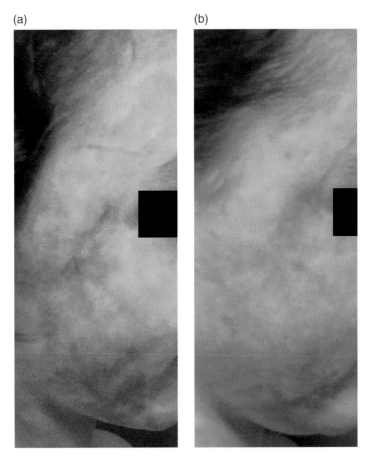

Figure 3.22 Hypopigmented scar after hot-water burn (a) 16 months post-trauma and (b) with better repigmentation one year post-needling combined with NCASCS. *Source:* Matthias Aust.

Figure 3.23 Hypopigmented scar after burn, lower back, 24 months post-trauma, before treatment. *Source:* Matthias Aust.

Figure 3.24 Improvement of the melanin level and thereby repigmentation of the scar one year post-treatment. *Source:* Matthias Aust.

(a) (b)

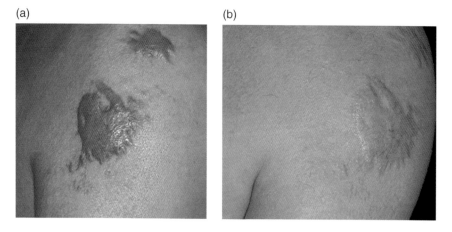

Figure 3.25 A post-burn keloid (a) is not the same as a true keloid and skin needling is a convenient way to treat these scars. The result seen (b) is after one year after a single session of 3 mm needling. *Source:* Matthias Aust.

Conclusion

Medical needling offers a new alternative treatment for burn scars by changing pathological scar collagen with thousands of micropunctures into a scar with normal collagen. When we prick skin, we puncture blood vessels and the release of platelets signals the release of growth factors which then improve dermal collagen, vascularization, and epidermal thickening. Medical needling liberates growth factors like VEGF and TGFß3, which initiate the replacement of parallel, packed scar collagen by physiological collagen I in a lattice orientation, with added elastin and glycosaminoglycans. The scars after medical needling tend to be smoother, softer, less itchy, and much less obvious. The skin becomes altogether more elastic and as a result contractures are also softened. In some cases, invasive surgery to treat contractures becomes unnecessary. Skin needling is showing us that it relieves tensions in tissues and minimizes the need for Z-plasty and major flaps. Early skin needling could help avoid scar contractures, which is one of the most crippling feature of burns. A significant problem arises for young girls as their breasts develop, because the breast tissue is entrapped by scar tissue and does not develop properly. Skin needling is worth doing for these patients and should be done as early as possible after the burn injury. There is good reason to believe that if we can change the spectrum of tissue healing dominated by TGFβ1 and -2 in the acute phase and convert it into a regenerative phase promoted by TGFβ3, we will have long-term effects and avoid contractures. Our experience at this stage is largely in treating well established burns, but the authors feel that skin needling should become a part of the early management of burn scars.

Repigmentation offers the ideal pretreatment for non-cultured autologous skin cell transplantation. Both treatments preserve the epidermis, which results in a reduced risk of new scarring or dyspigmentation.

Medical needling offers a treatment that, for the first time in medical history, can cause regeneration of tissue, soften burn scars, and reduce contractures. When done repeatedly and intensively the burn-scarred tissue can seem to be almost normal unscarred skin. However, the timing probably is of utmost importance. The authors believe skin needling should be done as soon after the burn injury as is reasonable because they have had experience treating burns within a few hours to days of the initial burn injury and it seems the earlier the needling, the greater the chance to heal with minimal scars.

Skin needling needs to be understood by clinicians treating burns so that this valuable technique can be offered to as many burn victims as possible.

References

1 Rawlins JM, Lam WL, Karoo RO, et al. Quantifying collagen type in mature burn scars: a novel approach using histology and digital image analysis. J Burn Care Res. 2006;27(1):60–65.

2 Roy D. Ablative facial resurfacing. Dermatol Clin. 2005;23(3):549–559,viii.

3 Avram MM, Tope WD, Yu T, et al. Hypertrophic scarring of the neck following ablative fractional carbon dioxide laser resurfacing. Lasers Surg Med. 2009;41(3):185–188.

4 Costa IM, Damasceno PS, Costa MC, Gomes KG. Review in peeling complications. J Cosmet Dermatol. 2017.

5 Aust MC, Fernandes D, Kolokythas P, et al. Percutaneous collagen induction therapy: an alternative treatment for scars, wrinkles, and skin laxity. Plast Reconstr Surg. 2008;121(4):1421–1429.

6 Fernandes D, Signorini M. Combating photoaging with percutaneous collagen induction. Clin Dermatol. 2008;26(2):192–199.

7 Aust MC, Bathe S, Fernandes D. Illustrated Guide to Percutaneous Collagen Induction: Basics, Indications, Uses. United Kingdom: Quintessence Publishing. 2013.

8 Camirand A, Doucet J. Needle dermabrasion. Aesthetic Plast Surg. 1997;21(1):48–51.

9 Orentreich DS, Orentreich N. Subcutaneous incisionless (subcision) surgery for the correction of depressed scars and wrinkles. Dermatol Surg. 1995;21(6):543–549.

10 Fernandes D. Percutaneous collagen induction: an alternative to laser resurfacing. Aesthet Surg J. 2002;22(3):307–9.

11 Aust MC, Knobloch K, Reimers K, et al. Percutaneous collagen induction therapy: an alternative treatment for burn scars. Burns : Journal of the International Society for Burn Injuries. 2010;36(6):836–843.

12 Aust MC, Reimers K, Kaplan HM, et al. Percutaneous collagen induction-regeneration in place of cicatrisation? J Plast Reconstr Aesthet Surg : JPRAS. 2011;64(1):97–107.

13 Aust MC, Reimers K, Gohritz A, et al. Percutaneous collagen induction. Scarless skin rejuvenation: fact or fiction? Clin Exp Dermatol. 2010;35(4):437–439.

14 El-Domyati M, Barakat M, Awad S, et al. Microneedling therapy for atrophic acne scars: an objective evaluation. J Clin Aesthet Dermatol. 2015;8(7):36–42.

15 El-Domyati M, Barakat M, Awad S, et al. Multiple microneedling sessions for minimally invasive facial rejuvenation: an objective assessment. Int J Dermatol. 2015;54(12):1361–1369.

16 Ferguson MW, O'Kane S. Scar-free healing: from embryonic mechanisms to adult therapeutic intervention. Philos Trans R Soc Lond B Biol Sci. 2004;359(1445):839–850.

17 Schultz GS, Wysocki A. Interactions between extracellular matrix and growth factors in wound healing. Wound Repair Regen. 2009;17(2):153–162.

18 Bandyopadhyay B, Fan J, Guan S, et al. A "traffic control" role for TGFbeta3: orchestrating dermal and epidermal cell motility during wound healing. J Cell Biol. 2006;172(7):1093–1105.

19 Occleston NL, Fairlamb D, Hutchison J, et al. Avotermin for the improvement of scar appearance: a new pharmaceutical in a new therapeutic area. Expert Opin Investig Drugs. 2009;18(8):1231–1239.

20 Aust MC, Reimers K, Repenning C, et al. Percutaneous collagen induction: minimally invasive skin rejuvenation without risk of hyperpigmentation-fact or fiction? Plast Reconstr Surg. 2008;122(5):1553–1563.

21 Aust MC, Reimers K, Kaplan HM, et al. Percutaneous collagen induction-regeneration in place of cicatrisation? J Plast Reconstr Aesthet Surg.

22 Aust MC, Reimers K, Kaplan HM, et al. Percutaneous collagen induction-regeneration in place of cicatrisation? J Plast Reconstr Aesthet Surg. 2010.

23 Yamaguchi Y, Hearing VJ. Melanocytes and their diseases. Cold Spring Harb Perspect Med. 2014;4(5).

24 Alam M, Warycha M. Complications of lasers and light treatments. Dermatol Ther. 2011;24(6):571–580.

25 Vaiyavatjamai P, Wattanakrai P. Side effects and complications of fractional 1550-nm erbium fiber laser treatment among Asians. J Cosmet Dermatol. 2011;10(4):313–316.

26 Aust MC, Reimers K, Repenning C, et al. Percutaneous collagen induction: minimally invasive skin rejuvenation without risk of hyperpigmentation-fact or fiction? Plast Reconstr Surg. 2008;122(5):1553–1563.

27 Onur E. The Treatment of Burn Scar Hypopigmentation and Surface Irregularity by Dermabrasion and Thin Skin Grafting. Plast Reconstr Surg. 1990.

28 Kahn AM, Cohen MJ. Treatment for depigmentation following burn injuries. Burns. 1996;22(7):552–554.

29 Cho S, Zheng Z, Park YK, Roh MR. The 308-nm excimer laser: a promising device for the treatment of childhood vitiligo. Photodermatology, Photoimmunology & Photomedicine. 2011;27(1):24–29.

30 Stoner M, Wood F. The treatment of hypopigmented lesions with cultured epithelial autograft. J Burn Care Rehabil. 2000;21:50–54.

31 Zhang DM, Hong WS, Fu LF, et al. A randomized controlled study of the effects of different modalities of narrow-band ultraviolet B therapy on the outcome of cultured autologous melanocytes transplantation in treating vitiligo. Dermatol Surg. 2014;40(4):420–426.

32 Ross EV, Naseef GS, McKinlay JR, et al. Comparison of carbon dioxide laser, erbium:YAG laser, dermabrasion, and dermatome. J Am Acad Dermatol. 2000;42(1):92–105.

33 Laws RA, Finley EM, McCollough ML, Grabski WJ. Alabaster skin after carbon dioxide laser resurfacing with histologic correlation. Dermatol Surg. 1998;24(6):633–636.

34 Bernstein LJ, Kauvar ANB, Grossman MC, Geronemus RG. The Short- and Long-Term Side Effects of Carbon Dioxide Laser Resurfacing. Dermatol Surg. 1997;23(7):519–525.

35 Thomas JR, Somenek M. Scar revision review. Arch Facial Plast Surg. 2012;14(3):162–174.

36 Busch KH, Bender R, Walezko N, et al. Combination of medical needling and non-cultured autologous skin cell transplantation (ReNovaCell) for repigmentation of hypopigmented burn scars. Burns. 2016;42(7):1556–1566.

4

Skin Care Used with Microneedling

Chytra V. Anand and
Parinitha Rao

Kosmoderma Clinics Bangalore, India

Introduction

Aging of the skin is undesirable and occurs with time due to both natural (intrinsic) and environmental (extrinsic) factors. Intrinsic factors include the unavoidable consequences of chronological aging, such as diminished levels of androgens and growth hormone, decreased collagen production, and breakdown of the elastin network. The extent of aging due to intrinsic factors is affected by genetic factors such as gender and ethnicity.

Extrinsic aging is predominately due to chronic exposure to damaging ultraviolet (UV) radiation, also known as photoaging. The effects of sunlight on the skin are estimated to account for up to 90% of visible skin aging. Histological studies have demonstrated significantly greater decreases in elastin and type I and type III collagen among sun-exposed individuals. Other extrinsic factors include psychological stress, diet, medications, smoking, air pollutants, and comorbid illness.

Together, intrinsic and extrinsic aging lead to facial skin attributes including fine lines, deep wrinkles, skin laxity, an increase in hyperpigmentation, reduced radiance, and an increase in visual and tactile roughness. To alleviate the signs of aging or to slow down the aging process, patients have incorporated skincare (cosmeceuticals) products into their daily routines, as well as undergone nonsurgical and noninvasive cosmetic procedures. Recently, it has been suggested that pairing skincare products or customizing skincare regimens with procedures can enhance patient results, reduce downtime, and enhance patient experience.

Skincare cosmeceutical products, such as antiaging moisturizers, have been shown to address intrinsic and extrinsic aging and reverse signs of aging.

Microneedling: Global Perspectives in Aesthetic Medicine, First Edition.
Edited by Elizabeth Bahar Houshmand.
© 2021 John Wiley & Sons Ltd. Published 2021 by John Wiley & Sons Ltd.

Microneedling is a cosmetic procedure gaining popularity as it has been clinically shown to address both intrinsic and extrinsic skin aging. This cosmetic procedure is minimally invasive and utilizes fine needles to puncture the skin, creating microwounds, which induces the release of growth factors and induction of collagen and elastin production [1].

Microneedling, also known as percutaneous collagen induction (PCI), has demonstrated efficacy for treating a variety of skin conditions, including atrophic acne scars, traumatic and burn scars, striae, and skin rejuvenation on all skin types.

Histological studies have shown that microneedling can tighten and improve the appearance of photoaged skin. This rejuvenation is associated with significant increases in collagen types I, III, and VII and elastin. The physical trauma caused by needle penetration induces the normal wound-healing response while causing minimal damage to the epidermis. A 400% increase in collagen and elastin has been demonstrated following several microneedling sessions [2]. Advantages of this procedure include simplicity, rapid recovery, being well tolerated, minimal risk of postinflammatory hyperpigmentation, convenience, and cost-effectiveness.

Microneedling has been further refined by combining it with radiofrequency (RF) technology. Insulated needles penetrate the skin, where radiofrequency currents produce thermal zones in the skin without damaging the overlying epidermis. This stimulates long-term dermal remodeling, neoelastogenesis, and neocollagenesis. The needle depth can be adjusted, which enables treatment of different layers of the dermis. Microneedling is also an effective method of enhancing the efficacy of chemical peels and other skin rejuvenation procedures [3].

As RF microneedling procedures continue to increase in popularity, it is important to study the use of a skincare regimens pre- and postprocedure.

Pre- and posttreatment skincare

Role of peptides

It has been predicted that skincare prior to a procedure "readies the skin, enhances metabolism for the trauma that is coming, revs up the machinery for repair, and adds the nutrients needed for repair" [4]. It is hypothesized that pairing an antiaging facial moisturizer with RF microneedling following a detailed skincare regimen should produce enhanced and optimal results to the patient, on both a short-term and a long-term basis. Additionally, although RF microneedling disrupts the barrier, the patient should tolerate the procedure with minimal side effects.

A clinical study was done to evaluate the tolerability and safety for use of a multi-ingredient antiaging moisturizer pre- and post-RF microneedling procedure, and to evaluate the improvement and conditioning of the facial skin using a multi-ingredient antiaging moisturizer for two weeks of twice-daily use prior to RF microneedling procedure and for four weeks of twice-daily use post-RF microneedling procedure. This multi-ingredient antiaging facial moisturizer was a comprehensive, all-in-one facial moisturizer that contains ingredients which specifically address aging in the epidermis, dermal-epidermal junction, and dermis [1].

The antiaging moisturizer was composed of the following key ingredients: astragalus membranaceus root extract, tetrahexyldecyl ascorbate (THD), ursolic acid, a blend of bioavailable peptides (including palmitoyl tripeptide-38), a blend of pure ceramides, natural cholesterol, fatty acids, and jojoba esters, sodium hyaluronate, and ubiquinone. The multi-ingredient antiaging formulation was enhanced to include a prebiotic ingredient, alpha glucan-oligosaccharide. The addition of this ingredient creates a robust, multitargeted antiaging moisturizer with the additional benefit of balancing and diversifying the skin microbiome. All other ingredients were maintained at efficacious levels.

A two-week run of DEJ face cream® (Revision Skincare®, Irving TX), a multi-ingredient antiaging face moisturizer, simultaneous to the washout period of all facial creams was performed. Patients were instructed to stop using topical astringents and abrasives for one week, antibiotics on the face for two weeks, retinoids (including retinol) on the face for two weeks, and glycolic or lactic acid for two weeks prior to the procedure. In addition, Gentle Cleansing Lotion, Revision Skincare®, a nonmedicated gentle cleanser, was dispensed to be utilized during the study [1].

Lastly, when excessive sun exposure was unavoidable, patients were directed to wear appropriate protective clothing and to use sunscreen lotion with SPF of 30 or higher. Patients were instructed to apply the DEJ face cream evenly to the face twice daily, once in the morning and once in the evening, two weeks prior to RF microneedling procedure, approximately 20 minutes after the RF microneedling procedure, and for four weeks postprocedure, with twice daily application.

Topical anesthetic cream was applied on the treatment area prior to RF microneedling. Before application of the anesthetic cream, patients were instructed to wash their faces thoroughly with lukewarm water and a cleanser. Patients were asked to apply DEJ face cream before leaving the office, approximately 20 minutes postprocedure. In this six-week open-label, single-site clinical study, 15 patients completed the study with no adverse events as evaluated by the investigator. At the end of the study, all tolerability parameters assessed by the investigator and patients were not significant compared to preprocedure.

Eighty percent of patients showed an improvement on the Glogau wrinkle scale, but improvement was not statistically significant between the baseline and end of study. Full-face skin evaluation was measured by the investigator at all visits and efficacy parameters included radiance, tone, smoothness, texture, redness, dryness, and overall appearance. Improvements in all skin attributes were statistically significant at the end of the study. Self-perceived skin attribute improvements were ranked as follows: overall improvement, brightness, texture, pigmentation, redness, and tightness. The combination of the antiaging facial moisturizer and RF microneedling was comfortable for the patients and patients were satisfied.

The results indicated that incorporation of specialty ingredients at efficacious levels produced statistically significant antiaging results. Furthermore, these ingredients were incorporated into the antiaging moisturizer because of their potential to target the layers of the skin susceptible to both intrinsic and extrinsic aging [1].

Another study was done to assess the safety and efficacy of two topical tri- and hexapeptide-containing products pre- and posttreatment with RF microneedling of the photoaged neck with respect to healing and aesthetic outcomes [3].

Novel topical products formulated using tri- and hexapeptide technology (TriHex Technology®) were used to clear the extracellular matrix, stimulate neocollagenesis and elastogenesis, decrease inflammation, and accelerate the epidermal healing process. Using this technology, a new product was developed to reduce post-treatment redness and discomfort associated with RF microneedling, to improve neocollagenesis and elastogenesis, and to improve skin hydration. The first skincare product (RSN; Regenerating Skin Nectar®; Alastin Skincare®, Inc.) was designed to be applied before and immediately following invasive and noninvasive aesthetic procedures to enhance elastin and collagen production for faster recovery and improved aesthetic outcomes.

The product was formulated with a proprietary TriHex Technology™, the flavanone naringenin, panthenyl triacetate, *Arnica montana* extract, and the carotenoids phytoene and phytofluene. The formulation possesses a high antioxidant activity to calm inflamed skin and reduce redness.

A second skincare product, Restorative Neck Complex (RNC; Restorative Neck Complex; Alastin Skincare®, Inc.) was a proprietary formulation which also incorporates TriHex Technology and a proprietary blend of peptides and potent antioxidants for treating crepey skin and photoaged discoloration of the neck and décolleté.

Each subject was instructed to cleanse their neck prior to applying the first product, RSN, in the morning and evening beginning two weeks prior to the RF microneedling procedure and continuing one week post-treatment. RSN was also applied to the neck within 15 minutes following RF microneedling. Beginning on the evening of study Day 21 (post-treatment Day 7), subjects applied the second product, RNC, morning and evening for the remainder of the study.

The results of the study showed that the mean Investigator Photodamage Assessment score was 2.3 at baseline, indicating moderately severe photodamaged skin prior to treatment. Mean scores steadily decreased, becoming significant at 30 days post-treatment, which persisted through Day 90. One subject observed wrinkle improvement using the RSN study product alone for the 14 days prior to the RF microneedling procedure. Based on mean Investigator Global Assessment scores, all skin quality parameters were statistically significantly improved by post-treatment Day 30.

The greatest changes occurred in tactile skin texture (79%), visual skin smoothness (62%), red, blotchy skin (62%), and overall appearance. Similar to Investigator Global Assessment scores, all 10 parameters in the Subject Skin Quality Questionnaire parameters showed improvements at post-treatment Day 30 which persisted until Day 90.

The RF microneedling procedure was well tolerated and no unexpected adverse events were reported. Subjective reports were mild or moderate and transient, being resolved within three to seven days. Similarly, objective reports of erythema and edema were mild and moderate, respectively, on the day of the procedure and resolved within three to seven days. There were no adverse events associated with the tri- and hexapeptide-containing test products.

The application of peptide-containing topical products has beneficial effects against the signs of intrinsic and extrinsic skin aging. These products rejuvenate the appearance of photoaged skin by clearing the extracellular matrix and stimulating collagen and elastin production. Overall, the results of this study provide additional evidence supporting the safety and efficacy of tri- and hexapeptide-containing topical products [3].

Role of growth factors

Growth factors (GFs) comprise a large group of regulatory proteins that attach to cell surface receptors and serve as chemical messengers. Via this interaction, they mediate inter- and intracellular signaling pathways that control cell growth, proliferation, and differentiation. Unlike hormones, the activity of GFs is confined to the vicinity of their sites of production. In the skin, GFs are synthesized by fibroblasts, keratinocytes, platelets, lymphocytes, and mast cells. Specific GFs regulate vital cellular activities, including mitogenesis, angiogenesis, chemotaxis, formation of the extracellular matrix (ECM), and control of other GFs.

When the skin is wounded, GFs accumulate at the site of injury and interact synergistically to initiate and coordinate wound healing. They can reverse the effects of collagenases, increase collagen levels, and decrease tissue inflammation.

Clinical studies have demonstrated that topical application of human- or animal-derived GFs or injection of autologous GFs may also increase dermal collagen synthesis, and that this is associated with reduced signs of skin aging such as fine lines and wrinkles. It is postulated that GFs can act synergistically to produce the desired effects. Topical GFs are derived from a variety of sources, including humans (epidermal cells, placental cells, foreskin, and colostrum), animals, plants, recombinant bacteria, and yeast [5].

Growth factors may be beneficial in reducing signs of skin aging owing to their ability to promote dermal fibroblast and keratinocyte proliferation and to induce extracellular matrix formation, including collagen. Endothelial precursor cells (EPCs), differentiated from human embryonic stem cell (hESC), have demonstrated their effects on the improvement of blood perfusion in damaged tissues.

Conditioned medium (CM) of hESC-derived EPC (hESC-EPC), which was composed of a large number of growth factors and cytokines, significantly improved signs of skin aging, and therefore could be one of the potential treatment options for skin rejuvenation. A 12-week randomized split-face study was undertaken to evaluate *in vivo* efficacy of microneedle fractional RF for skin rejuvenation in Asians, and furthermore the synergistic effect of stem cell conditioned medium (hESC-EPC CM) for skin rejuvenation.

Patients received three treatments each, spaced four weeks apart. Each patient's face was anesthetized using topical 4% lidocaine cream (LMX4, Ferndale Laboratories Inc., Ferndale, MI) about 30 minutes before the procedure. The face was cleansed with a mild soap and 70% alcohol. As per the manufacturer's recommendation, the full face was treated with a microneedle fractional RF device (Scarlet™, Viol Co., Korea). The treatment parameters were determined based on the specific anatomical location and proximity of underlying bones [6].

Treatment was delivered in a single, nonoverlapping pass over the indicated area. An epidermal cooling device (CARESYS, Danil SMC, Korea) was used to relieve pain and erythema after the treatment. Postoperatively, 1.5 ml of normal saline was painted for the fractional RF alone treatment side, and 1.5 ml of hESC-EPC CM was painted for the fractional RF plus hESC-EPC CM treatment sides. Patients were instructed to avoid washing their faces at least for one hour. *In vitro*, hESC-EPC CM significantly improved the proliferation and migration of dermal fibroblasts and epidermal keratinocytes and also increased collagen synthesis of fibroblasts.

Analysis of hESC-EPC CM with a multiplex cytokine array system indicated that hESC-EPCs secrete cytokines and chemokines such as EGF, bFGF, fractalkine, GM-CSF, IL-6, IL-8, PDGF-AA, and VEGF, which are well known to be important in normal angiogenesis and wound healing. It is well documented that hydrophilic molecules larger than 500 Dalton (Da) molecular weight have very low penetration through the stratum corneum. Most growth factors are large hydrophilic molecules greater than 20 kDa molecular weight; thus, penetration through the epidermis is an important matter to apply growth factors for skin rejuvenation.

In the study, microneedle fractional RF was conducted to enhance skin penetration of hESC-EPC CM, which creates 300-μm pin-hole wounds. It was confirmed that proteins in hESC-EPC CM could penetrate the epidermis directly when combined with microneedle fractional RF. It is expected that the presence of hESC-EPC CM in the dermis shows direct effects to dermal extracellular matrix and enhances wound healing following fractional RF.

The study demonstrated that combined treatment of microneedle fractional RF and hESC-EPC CM showed better results in patient satisfaction scores, investigator evaluations, skin roughness measured by Visiometer, and histologic increase of collagen than microneedle fractional RF–only treatment. It was concluded that microneedle fractional RF is a safe and effective treatment in Asian skin rejuvenation, and combined treatment of microneedle RF and stem cell conditioned medium showed a synergistic effect on skin rejuvenation [6].

Role of platelet-rich plasma

Skin needling efficacy depends on its capacity to induce neocollagenesis and the wound healing process in the upper dermis. Furthermore, skin needling provides a clear channel for topical agents to be absorbed more effectively through the top layer of the skin, such as the platelet-rich plasma (PRP).

PRP is defined as an autologous concentration of platelets in a small volume of plasma and it was initially developed in the 1970s. Plasma is rich in platelets, stem cells, and growth factors, and this stimulates the skin to produce more collagen. Platelets were thought to act exclusively with clotting. However, platelets also release many bioactive proteins responsible for attracting macrophages, mesenchymal stem cells, which not only promotes removal of necrotic tissue, but also enhances tissue regeneration and healing.

A split-face, prospective clinical trial was done, comparing skin needling followed by PRP treatment and skin needling treatment alone in patients with post-acne scarring. Thirty-five patients with post-acne scarring were included in the study. All the patients received four sequential treatments of skin microneedling using a dermaroller alone on the right side of the face, and skin microneedling followed by topical application of PRP on the left side of the face, with an interval of three weeks.

The area of interest was anesthetized using a thick application of topical anesthetic cream (EMLA) for about 30–45 minutes before the procedure. After preparation of the area with antiseptic and saline, the skin was stretched with one hand, and perpendicularly, rolling was done five times each in the horizontal, vertical, and oblique directions with the other hand. The treatment endpoint was identified as uniform pinpoint bleeding, which was easily controllable. Postprocedure, the area was cleansed with saline and ice packs were used for comforting the patient. Thereafter, the patient was advised to use a topical antibiotic, use sunscreen regularly, and follow sun-protective measures.

For PRP, 10 ml of autologous whole blood was collected into tubes containing acid citrate dextrose (ACD) and centrifuged at 2500rpm for 10 minutes in order to get PRP at the top of the test tube. Then, the PRP was further centrifuged at 3500 rpm for 10 minutes at room temperature of 22 degrees C in order to obtain a platelet-rich count. Platelet-poor plasma (PPP) was partly removed and partly used to resuspend the platelets. Calcium gluconate was added as an activator (1:9), i.e. 1 ml of calcium gluconate in 9 ml of PRP.

PRP is an autologous preparation of platelets in concentrated plasma, and contains a mixture of bioactive agents derived from both platelets and plasma. Various growth factors, including platelet-derived growth factor (PDGF), transforming growth factor (TGF), vascular endothelial growth factor (VEGF), and insulin-like growth factor (IGF), are secreted from the α-granules of concentrated platelets activated by aggregation inducer, which are very important in tissue remodeling, promoting connective tissue healing by upregulating collagen and protein synthesis. The study showed that there was a significant improvement of atrophic acne scars both on the side treated with skin needling alone (p values was < .001) as well as on the side treated with skin needling and PRP (p values was < .001); however, p values of comparing total results of both sides showed an insignificant difference denoting that both procedures gave comparably close results. Regarding patient satisfaction grades, there was a significant improvement after both treatment modalities, with insignificant differences between the two treatment modalities.

The patients experienced significantly less erythema and edema and less overall downtime in the side that was treated with skin needling and PRP as comparing to other side treated with skin needling alone. PRP was used for improving acne scars by increasing the healing mechanism, by accelerating tissue repair after skin needling, and by reducing adverse effects such as prolonged erythema [7].

Role of vitamin a and vitamin c

Vitamin A, a retinoic acid, is an essential vitamin (actually a hormone) for skin. It expresses its influence on 400–1000 genes that control proliferation and differentiation of all the major cells in the epidermis and dermis. Retinyl esters are the main form of vitamin A in the skin and for this reason topical vitamin A is applied in its ester forms (retinyl palmitate and retinyl acetate), with little use of retinol or retinoic acid directly. Vitamin C is also essential for the production of normal collagen. PCI and vitamin A switch on the fibroblasts to produce collagen and therefore increase the need for vitamin C.

Vitamin A may control the release of transforming growth factor (TGF)-3 in preference to TGF-1 and TGF-2 because, in general, retinoic acid seems to favor the development of a regenerative lattice-patterned collagen network rather than the parallel deposition of scar collagen found with cicatrization. TGFβ plays an enormous role in the first 48 hours of scar formation. Whereas TGFβ1 and TGFβ2 promote scar collagen, TGFβ3 seems to promote regeneration and scarless wound healing with a normal collagen lattice. The ideal treatment of scars should be to promote regeneration rather than cicatrization, and this could offer our patients the result they are hoping for [8].

Since it is well known that vitamins A and C are vital for production of new collagen and protection of existing collagen, it is not surprising that combining microneedling with topical antioxidants has been shown to enhance the regenerative process of microneedling-induced wound healing. Pretreatment priming of the skin with antioxidants may also serve to increase gene and protein expression responsible for skin regeneration. Caution is advised with concomitant use of topical products of any type during a microneedling procedure due to the risk of granuloma formation. In a case series published in 2014, three patients developed biopsy-proven foreign-body-type granulomas after the application of topical vitamin C during microneedling. Subsequent patch testing in these patients demonstrated a positive hypersensitivity to various chemicals within the topical vitamin C formulation [9].

The use of topical medications with or immediately after a microneedling procedure may increase the incidence of adverse effects because of the creation of channels within the epidermis and dermis that act as gateways into the body, allowing for the development of an immune response to immunogenic particles.

It is, thus, imperative to counsel patients on the avoidance of nonprescribed skincare products for the first week after the microneedling procedure as these may potentially induce a local or systemic hypersensitivity reaction. In addition, physicians need to use extreme caution when applying topical agents to the skin immediately after the microneedling session to avoid such complications [10].

General considerations: pretreatment, during treatment, and post-treatment

All patients may continue the use of any home skincare regimen (including retinoids, antioxidants, and growth factors) up until the time of the procedure. Oral anticoagulants do not need to be discontinued as the risk of uncontrollable bleeding during the microneedling treatment is negligible. Since the microneedling procedure is often used in combination with other treatments such as injections of hyaluronic acid filler and chemical peels and various dermatologic lasers, no "wash out" period is necessary before initiation of treatment. It is, however, recommended that for same-day treatments, the order of treatments be applied from deep to superficial (e.g. injectables before microneedling and/or laser irradiation) to maintain visual landmarks and prevent diffusion of injectables caused by tissue edema or bleeding.

Although any skin phototype can be treated, it is recommended that treatment be delayed in patients with a history of recent sun exposure (or who are visibly tanned) until all traces of suntan have faded, to avoid post-treatment dyspigmentation.

Meticulous skin preparation is important to decrease the risk of superficial skin infections. A gentle skin cleanser to remove makeup and debris from the skin's surface should be used before application of a topical anesthetic cream or gel to the treatment area. Typically a compounded 30% lidocaine cream (nonoccluded) is applied for 20 to 30 minutes, and removed with water-soaked gauze and alcohol prep immediately before the microneedling procedure.

When the clinical end point of uniform pinpoint bleeding has been achieved, ice water–soaked sterile gauze can be applied to remove excess blood. Treatment can then be pursued in an adjacent treatment area or quadrant. The use of tap water is discouraged because of its possible contamination with pathogenic organisms which could potentially increase the risk of infection in the treatment areas. If any bleeding persists after cleansing the treatment area, gentle pressure with dry sterile gauze should be applied for several minutes. A thin layer of hyaluronic acid gel can then be applied to the treatment region and allowed to dry.

For the first four hours after the procedure, the patient is instructed to apply the provided sample of hyaluronic acid gel to the skin. After four hours, a 1% hydro-cortisone cream or a nonallergenic moisturizing cream can be applied to the treatment regions two to four times daily for two to three days. The use of a nonchemical (or physical) sunblock with SPF 30 or higher is advocated (on top of the moisturizer) during the first post-treatment week. Application of makeup may be resumed two days after the procedure and any active skin care products that the patient used pretreatment can be resumed in five to seven days, when all traces of skin erythema have been resolved [10].

References

1 Zahr AS, Kononov T, Sensing W, et al. An open-label, single-site study to evaluate the tolerability, safety, and efficacy of using a novel facial moisturizer for preparation and accelerated healing pre and post a single full-face radiofrequency microneedling treatment. J Cosmet Dermatol. 2019. doi: 10.1111/jocd.12817

2 Aust MC, Fernandes D, Kolokythas P, et al. Percutaneous collagen induction therapy: an alternative treatment for scars, wrinkles, and skin laxity. Plast Reconstr Surg. 2008;121:1421–1429.

3 Gold MH, Sensing W, Biron JA. A topical regimen improves skin healing and aesthetic outcomes when combined with a radiofrequency microneedling procedure. J Cosmet Dermatol. 2019. doi: 10.1111/jocd.13037

4 Dayan SH, Waldrof H. The secret success factor, how skincare can enhance procedure outcomes exponentially. Modern Aesthetics. 2018:S3–S14.

5 Fabi S, Sundaram H. The potential of topical and injectable growth factors and cytokines for skin rejuvenation. Facial Plastic Surgery. 2014. doi: 10.1055/s-0034-1372423

6 Seo KY, Kim DH, Lee SE, et al. Skin rejuvenation by microneedle fractional radiofrequency and a human stem cell conditioned medium in Asian skin: a randomized controlled investigator blinded split-face study. J Cosmet Laser Ther. 2013. doi: 10.3109/14764172.2012.748201

7 Ibrahim MK, Ibrahim SM, Salem AM. Skin microneedling plus platelet-rich plasma versus skin microneedling alone in the treatment of atrophic post acne scars: a split face comparative study. Journal of Dermatological Treatment. 2018. doi: 10.1080/09546634.2017.1365111

8 Aust MC, Knobloch K, Reimers K, et al. Percutaneous collagen induction therapy: an alternative treatment for burn scars. Burns. 2010. doi: 10.1016/j.burns.2009.11.014

9 Soltani-Arabshahi R, Wong JW, et al. Facial allergic granulomatous reaction and systemic hypersensitivity associated with microneedle therapy for skin rejuvenation. JAMA Dermatol 2014;150: 68–72.

10 Alster TS, Graham PM. Microneedling: A Review and Practical Guide. Dermatol Surg. 2018. doi: 10.1097/DSS.0000000000001248

5 Treatment of Hyperpigmentation with Microneedling

Atchima Suwanchinda

School of Anti-aging and Regenerative Medicine, Mae Fah Luang University; Ramathibodi University Hospital, Mahidol University, Bangkok, Thailand

Key points

- Microneedling (MN) is an evolving treatment that has been studied in hyperpigmentation disorder.
- MN modalities can be effectively used as monotherapy or combination therapy.
- MN can be used as powerful drug-delivery treatment.
- MN carries a decreased risk of side effects compared to traditional skin resurfacing modalities. It offers greater safety than other modalities for patients with skin of color [Fitzpatrick skin types (FST) IV-VI].
- There is no evidence-based guideline presently established for the use of microneedling in treatment of hyperpigmentation

Introduction

Microneedling (MN), also known as percutaneous collagen induction (PCI) therapy, is a relatively new minimally invasive procedure involving superficial skin puncture by rolling multiple miniature fine needles into the skin [1]. In a short period of time, this procedure has gained popularity and acceptance in many treatment modalities as it is a simple, safe, cost-efficient, and effective technique with minimal training required [2]. It can be done on all skin types because it does not target specific chromophores in the skin and there is no thermal energy activation involvement. Therefore, MN has a minor effect on pigmentation. It decreases

Microneedling: Global Perspectives in Aesthetic Medicine, First Edition.
Edited by Elizabeth Bahar Houshmand.
© 2021 John Wiley & Sons Ltd. Published 2021 by John Wiley & Sons Ltd.

the risks for postinflammatory hyper/hypopigmentation (PIH) and dyspigmentation compared to traditional skin resurfacing modalities, including lasers, dermabrasion, and chemical peels [3, 4]. The risks of infection and scarring are relatively low in MN procedures compared to traditional ones because MN keeps the epidermis partially intact and the remaining skin barrier accelerates the recovery healing phase [3, 5]. Because of MN carries a decreased risk of these potential complications, it becomes a favorable treatment in patients with skin of color (Fitzpatrick skin types (FST) IV-VI) [3].

MN has been reported as a successful treatment modality for many dermatologic conditions such as skin rejuvenation, rhytids, striae, active acne, acne scaring, surgical scaring, enlarged pores, androgenic alopecia, alopecia areata, primary hyperhidrosis, striae distensae, and transdermal drug delivery [2, 4, 6, 7]. Furthermore, pigmentations including melasma and periorbital hypermelanosis are among the indications that have gained a lot of attention recently [8–12]. Apart from dermatologic and aesthetic conditions, MN has been explored for other modalities, including photodynamic therapy, allergy testing, biological fluid sampling, and vaccination [13–15].

Principle and mechanism of action of microneedling

The basic principle of MN procedures is the repetitive application of the device with needles of length between 0.5 and 1.5 mm on the skin, with multiple directions to generate transient epidermal and dermal pores ranging from 25 to 3,000 μm in depth in order to upregulate normal skin synthesis and minimize the risk of inflammation or trauma which may produce fibrosis [16]. The range of MN devices has expanded in recent years and now includes powered pens and rollers, with microneedles ranging in length from 0.25 to 3.0 mm [17]. After an MN procedure, the generation of microchannels induces a skin injury with slight epidermal damage and stimulates the dermal wound healing cascade, including inflammation, proliferation, and remodeling. As a result, many growth factors are released, such as platelet-derived growth factor (PDGF), fibroblast growth factor (FGF), transforming growth factor alpha (TGFα) and transforming growth factor beta (TGFβ) [18, 19]. Neocollagenesis, elastin synthesis, and neovascularization occur due to fibroblast proliferation and migration [1, 20, 21]. A fibronectin network is generated five days after injury, providing a deposition of type III collagen that is ultimately replaced by collagen type I over weeks to months, contributing to skin tightening clinically as well as scar and rhytids reduction [18, 22]. The 500–600 μm depth of 1.5 mm–length needles is suitable for induce neocollagenesis [2]. There is also upregulation of glycosaminoglycans

(GAGs) and diverse growth factors such as vascular endothelial growth factor (VEGF), epidermal growth factor (EGF), and FGF-7 [18, 19]. Aust et al. also demonstrated that TGFβ3 is upregulated, which encourages regeneration and scarless wound healing. The ratio of TGFβ3 to TGFβ1 and TGFβ2, the latter being responsible for fibrotic scaring, may partly explain the beneficial basis of MN procedure [19].

Aust et al. have studied histological examination after four sessions of MN with a monthly interval. They showed that, at the treated areas, there was a 400% increase in collagen and elastin deposition at six months postprocedure, with a stratum spinosum thickening and normal rete ridges at one-year follow-up. The treated area appeared to have a normal lattice pattern rather than parallel bundles as observed in scar tissue [5].

This MN treatment can be used on its own and combined with topical products as an augmented transdermal drug delivery system through these micropores in the stratum corneum [23, 24]. Many products are used, such as platelet-rich plasma (PRP) and human embryonic stem cell–derived endothelial precursor cell conditioned medium (hESC-EPC CM), providing extra growth factors to enrich collagen production, while other agents, such a minoxidil, depigmenting serum, and tranexamic acid enhance their penetration and increase clinical efficacy [24]. It also can combine with radiofrequency through fractional radiofrequency (FRF), creating thermal injury to the dermis and inducing new collagen synthesis [6, 24]. This chapter will focus on microneedling of hyperpigmentation problems through different mechanisms.

Hyperpigmentation

In normal skin, the melanocytes are scattered among the basal cell keratinocytes with the ratio of 1:10 along the dermoepidermal interface [25, 26]. The melanocytes do not keratinize, but their main function is to synthesize, deposit, and transport melanin pigments to nearby keratinocytes through melanosomes, the unique intracytoplasmic organelle within melanocytes. Melanin absorbs UV waves to prevent keratinocytes' DNA damage [27]. The number of epidermal melanocytes is very stable. The major determinant of normal skin color is the activity of the melanocytes, such as the quality and quantity of melanin production, not the density of the melanocytes. However, proliferation of melanocytes can occur under specific conditions. There are limited hyperpigmented conditions in the literature which have been experimented with using MN treatment. Melasma and periorbital melanosis have been published, showing various improvement [28]. These two hyperpigmented conditions will be further elaborated in this chapter.

Melasma

Melasma is one of the most common acquired symmetrical hypermelanotic disorders, mostly affecting females with darker skin types [29]. It has a considerable negative psychological impact on the patient's quality of life [30]. Managing melasma is still a difficult challenge due to inconsistent treatment results and frequent recurrence despite successful clearance. Melasma is classified as epidermal, dermal, and mixed type based upon the primary location of melanin. Recent studies revealed that melasma is now considered to be a complex interaction between various cells, including epidermal melanocytes, keratinocytes, dermal fibroblasts, mast cells, vascular endothelial cells, and sebocytes [31]. It is also thought to be a photoaging skin disorder [32]. Many factors trigger melasma, such as sun exposure, genetic influences, hormones (e.g. elevated levels of estrogens and progesterone, pregnancy, contraceptive pill, and hormone replacement therapy), thyroid abnormalities, drugs (e.g. Dilantin, antimalarial drugs, tetracycline, minocycline), malnutrition (e.g. B12 deficiency), inflammation, and reactive oxygen species [30, 33, 34]. Histological changes in melasma are evident in the epidermis, dermis, and extracellular matrix. Apart from epidermal pigmentation, which was significantly increased in all epidermal layers even in the stratum corneum, its histologic findings include basement membrane thinning and disruption. Antibody to collagen type IV immunostaining shows disruption to the basal membrane in melasma skin, resulting in facilitating melanocytes and melanin migration to the dermis [35]. The ultrastructure of melasma skin also showed that the amount of cytoplasmic organelles (e.g. melanosome, mitochondria, microvesicles, endoplasmic reticulum, and Golgi apparatus) inside basal keratinocytes and melanocytes were greater, and there was higher structural damage manifested by disruptions, gaps, thinning, and lower density of lamina densa and loss of anchoring fibrils in lower lamina lucida [36]. Other histologic features in melasma skin included prominent solar elastosis, significant increased number of mast cells infiltration located particularly around elastotic area of melasma skin, increased melanophages and free melanin in the dermis, and a significant increase in number of blood vessels, vessel size, and vessel density [35, 37–40]. Sebocytes also produce growth factors and cytokines to exert paracrine effects on melanocytes. These histologic features of melasma strongly suggest that melasma should not be considered only a disease of melanocytes, but rather a complex interaction between various cells. This complicated pathogenesis of melasma leads to difficult management and is likely to recur post-treatment.

Currently, many therapeutic options are available for melasma treatment. These modalities include topical, oral, procedural, and combination treatment. Each one is aimed at diverse aspects of the pathogenesis of melasma, consisting of pigmentation, inflammation, vascularity, and photodamage [41]. Topical depigmenting agents, including photoprotection, are typically used as the main therapy for melasma. The most common agent use is hydroquinone (HQ), which inhibits melanin production through competitive inhibition of tyrosinase, and prevents the conversion of DOPA to melanin [42]. However, concomitant use of different topical therapies with various mechanisms of action should be considered more than monotherapy. MN was investigated as a possible treatment for melasma due to its advantage of avoiding the risks of pigmentation changes when compared to other therapeutic alternatives, including dermabrasion, laser treatment, and chemical peelings [3, 28, 43]. This procedure offers a higher safety profile in the skin of patients of color [3].

Microneedling in melasma

There is no evidence-based guideline presently established for the use and efficacy of MN on melasma patients. There are various protocols with inconsistent progression. In daily clinical practice, this MN treatment has been used with a variety of approaches depending on physician preferences. Despite the aforementioned fact, clinical improvement has been observed with the use of both MN alone and as a drug-delivery enhancement. It is also a common use in the population of people of color for the treatment of hyperpigmentation disorder.

A quasiexperimental study by Cassiano et al. demonstrated the early histological changes of the MN effects alone on melasma. Seven days after one session with 1.5 mm–length microneedles, there was a significant reduction in melanin density, pendulous melanocytes, and basement membrane damage. It also induced slight epidermal hyperplasia, fibroblast proliferation, subepidermal deposition of GAGs and fibrin, neocollagenesis, and increase in Ki67 marked keratinocytes – which means that MN has promoted early changes in the epidermis and upper dermis, leading to the reversal of some structural modifications in melasma. In addition, this modified environment disfavors the contact of melanocytes with dermal released melanogenic stimuli such as stem-cell factor, endothelin-1, and hepatocytes growth factor [11]. Other histological findings were shown in a pilot study of six recalcitrant melasma patients. Among those with more than five years of disease evolution that has relapsed after at least three attempts at treatment, the histopathology between baseline treatment to 15 days after two sessions at 30-day interval with 1.5 mm–length microneedles treatment demonstrated that all cases have epithelium thickening, epithelial melanin pigmentation reduction, upper dermis collagen densification ($p = 0.03$), and basement membrane restoration. The clinical evaluation showed a significant reduction in Melasma Area and Severity Index (MASI) score, Melasma Quality of Life Scale (MELASQoL),and increase in luminance colorimetric value ($p < 0.03$). All patients were followed for six months with use of daily broad-spectrum sunscreen and triple combination (Tri-Luma, Galderma) application, without relapse [10].

MN combination treatments have also been evidenced to aid the improvement of treatment of recalcitrant melasma. The combination treatment study was conducted in 22 melasma patients, who were unresponsive to topical lightening agents and sunscreen, with two sessions of 1.5 mm–length microneedles, 30-day interval. The treatment was performed with back-and-forth movements, about 10 times in each of four different directions, resulting in diffuse erythema and discrete punctuated bleeding. Every patient was instructed to use depigmenting agent 0.05% tretinoin + 4% hydroquinone + 1% fluocinolone acetonide and sunscreen with SPF 60 daily starting 24 hours post-procedure. There were no serious side effects and the treatment was well tolerated. All patients were responsive to the treatment and reported satisfaction with the results [9].

A split-face trial of 16 women with recalcitrant dermal- or mixed-type melasma was conducted to compare two treatments: (i) using the combination of the low-fluence 1064 nm Q-switched neodymium-doped yttrium aluminum garnet (QS-Nd:YAG) laser with vitamin C (Redoxan-C™) and 1.5 mm and 0.5 mm–length microneedles (Dermapen™) for cheeks and periorbital areas, respectively, on one side of the face, and (ii) using QS-Nd:YAG 1,064 nm alone on the other side of the face – both for a series of four monthly treatments. The evaluations showed that the combination treatment group has a significantly lower mean MASI score and better treatment response while the adverse effects and recurrence rates were no different. It was suggested that the QS-Nd:YAG laser increased blood circulation in the dermis, resulting in an enhancement of the mechanical effect of MN to promote vitamin C penetration [12].

Enhancing the drug delivery effect is also a common purpose for melasma treatment, particularly in skin of color [3]. The stratum corneum, which is the outermost layer of the epidermis, serves as a major role in this application. It ranges from 10 to 20 microns in thickness and consists of a semipermeable laminated surface aggregation of keratinized squamous epithelial cells embedded in an intercellular lipid matrix of mainly fatty acids, cholesterol, cholesterol sulfate, and ceramides [44]. Its function serves as a physiologic barrier to microbiologic invasion and chemical penetration from the environment, as well as a barrier to fluid and solution. As the result, the stratum corneum is the main barrier to the drugs' percutaneous absorption and significantly restricts the drugs' transdermal delivery. Therefore, drug molecules must be low molecular weight and/or small in size as well as be lipophilic molecules due to their deeper penetration than hydrophilic ones [45, 46]. Many skin penetration enhancement techniques have been developed to improve transdermal drug delivery, physically or chemically, including electroporation, sonophoresis, and iontophoresis, which support the stratum corneum layer permeability [47–50]. Drugs and agents can be applied topically after channels are created by microneedling or can be simultaneously infused during microneedling (DermaFrac™ device, Genesis Biosystems) [3].

Various depigmenting agents have been used, such as vitamin C, antiaging serum, rucinol, sophora-alpha, and tranexamic acid. Theoretically, vitamin C interacts with copper ions at the tyrosinase-active site, resulting in inhibiting the tyrosinase enzyme and thereby reducing melanin synthesis [51]. Tranexamic acid (TA) is a plasmin inhibitor that prevents fibrinolysis and reduces blood loss. Its primary used for melasma treatment was described by Nijor in 1979 [52, 53]. Tranexamic acid is a synthetic lysine derivation and exerts its effect by blocking the plasminogen-lysine binding site reversibly, thus inhibiting the plasminogen activator from converting plasminogen to plasmin [54]. Plasminogen exists in human epidermal basal cells and can be induced by ultraviolet radiation, leading to melanogenesis. According to the antiplasmin activity of tranexamic acid, it inhibits melanin synthesis by decreasing the level of alpha-melanocyte stimulating hormone (α-MSH) [41].

Tranexamic acid also has a similar structure to tyrosine, thereby competitively inhibiting the tyrosinase enzyme activity [9]. Furthermore, one study has shown that tranexamic acid can reduce the levels of endothelin-1 and VEGF, which causes the vascularity in melasma [41, 55]. Various routes of administration, including oral, topical, and intradermal microinjections of tranexamic acid, have been studied as a treatment for melasma, with successful results [54, 56–58]. However, the mechanism of skin lightening via MN is not yet well established.

Ismail et al. conducted a study of 30 female melasma patients, with six treatments of MN with vitamin C transdermal delivery every two weeks [59]. A dermaroller with 540 fine titanium microneedles of 1.5 mm length was rolled about 10 passes in each direction or until pinpoint bleeding was shown. A 20% pure L-Ascorbic acid from Fusion Mesotherapy Company was applied immediately after the MN procedure. All patients were instructed to use regular sunscreen with sun protective factor of at least 50 and to avoid going out in strong sunlight. The results showed that every patient had improved clinically at the end of sessions. The MASI score decreased significantly compared to the last session ($p < 0.0001$).

A comparison split-face study by Fabbrocini et al. on the combination treatment of MN using a dermaroller with 0.5 mm–length microneedles plus depigmenting serum (containing rucinol and sophora-alpha) versus the depigment serum alone was conducted in 20 patients (FST II-V). The results achieved after two sessions with one-month interval were assessed. The side of the face that received the combination treatment of MN and depigmenting serum exhibited erythema and swelling for a few days. No serious side effect was reported. At the first treatment, each patient was instructed to use the home dermaroller (Dermaroller™ Model C8, 0.13 mm) on the combination side of the face and then apply a standardized amount of the depigmenting serum immediately once a day, every day for two months to achieve better results. Broad-spectrum sunscreen was applied routinely on the whole face. The result showed that combined-treatment side had a statistically significant reduction in MASI score and luminosity index (L) measured by spectrocolorimeter compared to the side treated with depigmenting serum monotherapy alone. The clinical symptoms were significantly improved [60].

Another randomized controlled trial conducted by Budamakuntla et al. was done to compare the tranexamic acid microinjections alone to the combination treatment of MN and tranexamic acid in 60 patients (FST IV-V) with moderate to severe melasma. The procedure was done three times with a four-week interval and followed up for three consecutive months. The result showed a 44.41% improvement in MASI scores in the combined MN group compared with 35.72% improvement in MASI scores in the microinjection-alone group. Furthermore, at the last follow up more than 50% clinical improvement was shown in 26.09% of patients in the microinjections group, compared with 41.38% of patients in the combined-MN group [61]. No adverse effects were reported in this study.

All the studies showed favorable outcomes with the combination modalities. Adverse effects included mild discomfort, burning sensation, itching, transient erythema, and edema [23, 24, 28]. However, in all these studies there was a discrepancy in treatment protocol, microneedle devices, needle size, applied formulation, and pre- and post-care treatment, which possibly affected the clinical outcomes [62].

Periorbital melanosis

Periorbital melanosis presents with dark circles under both eyes occurring after puberty or in early childhood. It has multifactorial pathogenesis, including genetic predisposition, dermal melanocytosis, postinflammatory pigmentation secondary to atopic or allergic contact dermatitis, excessive or superficial location of vasculature, hormonal abnormalities, pigmentary demarcation lines, shadowing due to skin laxity, and tear troughs associated with aging [63–65]. It is commonly found in dark-skinned patients, especially Asians. This condition is a cosmetic concern for many patients, as it gives a sad or tired look [66]. Many treatment modalities have been tried with variable success, including topical agents [67], chemical peels [68], laser treatment [69], and fat grafts [70]. None of these treatments give consistent effective results [71].

Microneedling in periorbital melanosis

Microneedling therapy has shown success in treatment of periorbital melanosis. There was a one case report of male patient (FST V) using the combination of 0.25 mm MN with simultaneous vacuum-assisted serum infusion of active ingredients and DermaFrac treatment, which included antiaging serum (containing myristoyl pentapeptide 17 sympeptide, acetyl octapeptide-3 SNAP8, palmitoyl pentapeptide-4matrixyl, acetyl hexapeptide-8 argirilene, and tripeptide syn-ake) and whitening serum (containing kojic acid). Per the Physician Global Assessment scale, there was 50–75% improvement after four sessions and 75–90% improvement after 12 sessions [71]. There were no side effects described in this study. The author postulated that the improvement may be secondary to the better skin hydration and the induction of new collagen and elastin synthesis may have lessened the visibility of dermal pigment [71]. Another study report of the combination of MN and 10% trichloroacetic acid (TCA) peels in 13 patients were explored using automatic 0.5–1 mm–length microneedles of the microneedle therapy system Handhold (AMTS-H – Mcure Co., Ltd) followed by topical application of 10% TCA solution to each infraorbital area for five minutes. Almost all patients (92.3%) showed significant improvement (fair or better) on both physician and patient global assessment. There was no recurrence at four months [66]. Transient side effects, including mild discomfort, edema, and erythema, were reported. No hyperpigmentation, hypopigmentation, or scarring was observed during monthly follow-up [66]. In this study, even the low TCA concentration could reach the dermis because TCA molecules penetrate fast (due to their very lipophilic nature) after the increased epidermal permeability from MN [72].

Microneedling with biological agents for hyperpigmentation disorder

Topical biological agents used with MN include platelet-rich plasma (PRP), acellular extracted growth factors, stem cell–targeted small proteins, cultured or extracted bone marrow–derived mesenchymal cells [73], and small peptides that target existing banks of quiescent stem cells [74]. None are FDA approved for this purpose, due to the difficulty in measuring efficacy of these treatments – including the differences in the manufacturing and processing of these biological proteins, which affect the efficacy [74]. Currently, no published studies address the potential toxicity of these topical agents applied to skin treated with either MN or thermal needling [74].

The uptake of these drugs through damaged skin can be upward of 10 times the systemic concentration over drugs taken orally or applied to intact skin [74]. The study done by Haak et al. demonstrated the increased uptake of dermaceutical compounds after MN [75]. Kalluri et al. also showed that nonthermal microchannels close at about four to five hours postinjury, when a fibrin plug is formed [76, 77]. Although nonthermal needling channels close after several hours, thermal needling creates an injury similar to a subepidermal sponge, according to Oleson et al. [77]. The vehicle type of the topical agent directly affects the degree of uptake. Gel-like substances are somewhat inhibited due to their physical properties, whereas thinner liquids seem to be better absorbed [74, 77].

Microneedling with platelet-rich plasma (PRP)

PRP is developed by enriching plasma with an autologous high concentration of platelets derived from whole blood [17, 78]. Normal platelet levels in blood range from 150,000 to 400,000 platelets/μl or 150 to 400 × 109/L. PRP is targeted to prepare a platelet count greater than 1,000,000 platelets/μl, based on the studies showing the level of healing enhancement in bone and soft tissue [79]. Most of the PRP preparations in today's market provide a concentration that is four to eight times higher than that of peripheral blood [80].

PRP has multiple uses in dermatology, such as for androgenic alopecia, scar revision, acne scarring, skin rejuvenation, dermal augmentation, striae distensae, skin aging, wrinkles, melasma and dyspigmentation, hair transplantation surgery, and periocular circles [81]. Even though, up to date, our knowledge regarding the PRP mechanism in melasma improvement is limited, there is clinical evidence in favor of using PRP as a new therapeutic option in melasma. Several studies addressed the therapeutic effect of PRP in melasma treatment – either monotherapy or combination with other modalities [82–84]. Recently, there was a randomized, split-face, single-blinded prospective pilot study in 10 female Asian (Thai) patients with bilateral mixed-type melasma. The subjects underwent four treatment sessions every two weeks, with intradermal PRP injections on one side of the face (PRP condition) and normal saline on the other (control condition). The PRP injection side significantly improved melasma within six weeks in terms of modified MASI (mMASI) scores, patient satisfaction, and Antera®-assessed melanin levels. Side effects of treatment were mild and resolved spontaneously within a few days [85].

In Asia, Melasma is one of the most common skin disorders in daily practice. Its recalcitrant nature makes it difficult to overcome. With clinical evidence of the efficacy of using PRP in melasma together with the benefits of MN on Asian skin, this combination forms a great duo to auspiciously tackle melasma. (See Figure 5.1.)

The attractive component of PRP is its high concentration of growth factors [17]. PRP may act through a degranulation of the α-granules. There are more than 30 bioactive substances in these granules [86]. Upon platelet activation, many growth factors are released, such as epidermal growth factor (EGF), transforming growth factor beta (TGFβ), and platelet-derived growth factors (PDGF). These factors helps to regulate the proliferation and the differentiation of effector cells [87]. TGFβ aids in basement membrane healing by laminin, collagen IV, and tenascin. Both EGF and TGFβ1 inhibit melanin synthesis. TGFβ1 has an effect on melanogenesis by the reduction of the activity of tyrosinase and microphthalmia-associated transcription factor (MITF) promoter, plus decreased tyrosinase-related protein production. Moreover, TGFβ delays the activation of extracellular signal-regulated kinase (ERK) at six hours instead of in minutes like other growth factors [88]. Lastly, TGFβ also can inhibit the expression of paired-box homeotic

(a)   (b)

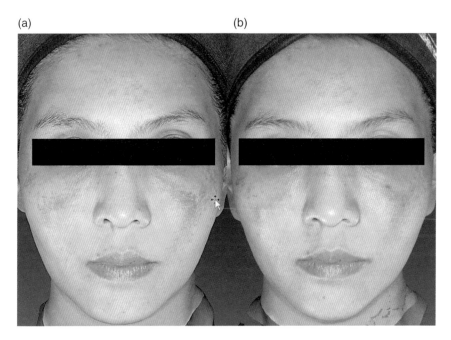

Figure 5.1 (a) Before treatment picture of mixed type melasma in 39-years old Thai female patient. (b) After 3-weeks treatment picture of same patient after one session of the combination of microneedling treatment with platelet-rich plasma (PRP). Moderate improvement was shown. (3D LifeViz® Mini, *Quantificare*, Valbonne, *France*). *Source:* Anchalee Srinakorn.

gene (PAX 3), which is a key regulator of UV-induced melanogenesis [89]. EGF decreases melanogenesis by inhibiting PGE2 and tyrosinase [90]. PDGF stimulates collagen synthesis and the extracellular components, particularly hyaluronic acid, leading to increase in skin volume by increasing the formation of blood vessels, collagen, and components of the extracellular matrix, including hyaluronic acid [90]. When the volume of the skin increases, it may obscure the dyspigmentation, showing more glowing skin [90]. Several studies have demonstrated that there is a significantly higher regression in epidermal hyperpigmentation than mixed type with PRP treatment [82]. A lower percentage of improvement in the higher Fitzpatrick skin phototype (V) and the more resistant mixed type of melasma have been found [83, 84, 91].

Hofny et al. studied the comparison of PRP delivery through MN using a dermapen versus microinjections using mesoneedles. The study demonstrated an excellent improvement by a significant decrease in the baseline MASI and mMASI scores in both epidermal and mixed types of melasma following PRP treatment, with no significant difference in the degree of improvement between the two application approaches [84].

There was one report of the study using the autologous human platelet rich fibrin (PRF-L) for exogenous ochronosis (EO). Three cases of EO were treated with a split-face approach, where PRF-L was applied right before MN treatment on one side and intradermal injections were administered on the other side. The treatment was done every two weeks for eight weeks. The improvement was measured with a 10-point grading scale and dermoscopic examination, plus a five-point grading scale to assess patient satisfaction. All three patients demonstrated significant improvement and were very satisfied in the fourth week of treatment [92].

Microneedling with cell-based therapies and stem cell conditioned medium

Cell-based therapies using one's own body's stem cells and growth factors for repairing damaged tissue and skin rejuvenation are emerging as innovative antiaging treatments, and the development of targeted peptides or small proteins to stimulate the existing stem cells has also been explored since 2015. Even though the use of adipose-derived stem cells (ADSCs) has been restricted by federal regulations in most countries, some Asian countries have been using ADSCs for skin rejuvenation and treatment of hyperpigmentation.

Stem cells may have a benefit on tissue regeneration through complex paracrine effects in addition to their proposed direct cellular mechanism [93]. Furthermore, stem cells themselves synthesize and secrete a variety of growth factors, cytokines, extracellular matrix proteins, and other bioactive proteins that help in tissue regeneration and healing processes, including regulating the function of individual stem cells [93, 94]. Animal studies in mice from China have demonstrated that the transplanted bone marrow–derived mesenchymal stem cells (BM-MSCs) differentiate into functional cells and play paracrine roles to recruit more endogenous cells for tissue remodeling in the initial stage of wound healing [73]. Recently, topical bone marrow–derived stem cells from multiple sources has been reported [74]. Mesenchymal stem cells from adipose tissue, ADSCs, show multi-lineage developmental plasticity and are similar to bone marrow–derived mesenchymal stem cells (BM-MSCs) with respect to surface markers and gene profiling [95]. Additionally, both stem cell types produce and secrete various cytokines, such as vascular endothelial growth factor (VEGF), hepatocyte growth factor, and transforming growth factor (TGF), which are the key stem cell functions exhibiting diverse pharmacological actions [95]. Particularly, TGFβ has a well-documented role in the regulation of melanocytic homeostasis [96]. Due to its abundance and own body's cells, ADSCs have been shown to be a promising source for regenerative clinical application. They have also been used in disorders of pigmentation.

The rationale of using ADSCs)in hyperpigmentation was based on a report of its whitening effect using in vitro culture approaches [95]. There is interaction between epidermal melanocytes and stromal cells regulating the skin pigmentation. Jeon et al. evaluated the effect of ADSCs on UVB-irradiated mouse skin, which demonstrated that there was a suppression of skin pigmentation and reduction of skin thickness following UVB irradiation in the ADSCs-injected side of the face in this split-face study. The tyrosinase activity and melanin content of the ADSCs-injected side were significantly reduced [97]. Klar et al. reported that substituting ADSCs for dermal fibroblasts alters pigmentation of engineered skin grafts [98]. This study highlighted the negative influence of adipose mesenchymal cells on the pigmentary compartment within skin equivalents, even with sufficient epithelial regeneration [98]. Additionally, it showed that melanocytes responded to the increased levels of TGFβ1 by downregulating the tyrosinase enzyme, which leads to decreased melanin synthesis and reduction in pigmentation [98]. TGFβ signaling has been shown to play a crucial role in controlling melanocyte stem cell return to quiescence in the early anagen phase of the hair follicle cycle [99]. The quiescent state includes suppression of MITF and its melanogenic targets. The ADSCs-derived TGFβ acts as an antagonist to melanocytic differentiation and could responsible for the hypopigmentary effects [99].

Conditioned media (CM) from cultured adipose mesenchymal cells (ADSC-CM) has been used for skin rejuvenation. A study by Kim et al. revealed the inhibition of the melanin synthesis and tyrosinase activity in a dose-dependent pattern with ADSC-CM treatment in B16 melanoma cells. The results of this study indicated that secretory factors of ADSC inhibit melanin synthesis by downregulating the expression of tyrosinase and TRP1, which are mainly mediated by TGFβ1 [95]. The hESC-EPC CM was reported in inhibition of the melanogenesis in B16 melanoma cells demonstrating the whitening effects [94, 100]. This biologic substance could lead to improvement in abnormal pigmentation. The hESC-EPC CM helps increase wound tensile strength and speed the process of wound healing by significantly enhancing the migration and proliferation of dermal fibroblasts and epidermal keratinocytes and increasing collagen synthesis [94, 101]. In vitro, It has been shown that hESC-EPCs also secrete high level of growth factors, cytokines, and chemokines such as EGF, bFGF, fractalkine, GM-CSF, IL-6, IL-8, PDGF-AA, and VEGF, which are important in normal angiogenesis and wound healing [94, 101]. Their pharmacological actions significantly improved the proliferation and migration of dermal fibroblasts and epidermal keratinocytes and increased collagen synthesis [101]. These properties could lead to antiaging effects [102]. However, most of these growth factors are large hydrophilic molecules greater than 20 kDa while hydrophilic molecules larger than 500 Da have poor penetration to the stratum corneum [103]. The MN procedure enhancing skin penetration could be one alternative to bring these growth factors into the dermis to create pharmacological effects.

A 12-week double-blind randomized controlled split-face study by Lee et al. investigated the effects of the secretory factors of hESC-EPC on aged skin in 25 Asian women. Each side of the face was randomly allocated to hESC-EPC CM or saline. A 0.25-mm microneedle roller was used to enhance penetration.

Five treatment sessions were repeated at two-week intervals. The Physician Global Assessment of pigmentation and wrinkles after the treatment showed statistically significant improvement on the side that received a combination of MN and hESC-EPC CM compared to MN alone (p<0.05). Mexameter® and Visiometer® also revealed statistically significant effects of MN and hESC-EPC CM on both pigmentation and wrinkles (p<0.05). The side effects were minimal; mild desquamation was reported in one patient [94]. This study demonstrated the efficacy of the soluble factors of stem cells on skin rejuvenation in vivo. Conditioned media from cultured adipose mesenchymal cells also suppressed expression of melanocytic genes. The study demonstrated the decreased numbers of MITFþ melanocytes in dermal equivalents when ASCs are included. There was a diminished expression of the differentiated melanocytic factors tyrosinase, TRP1, and Sox9. The melanocyte antagonists exhibited strong expression of TGFβ1 by these cells [94].

Microneedling technical and clinical considerations

Devices

Nonthermal MN devices come in three main types: stamps, rollers, and motorized pens. Each type has its own advantages and disadvantages The original dermal roller devices comprise evenly distributed needles affixed to a drum-shaped roller [74]. There is different needle size which operators can choose to match skin pathology.

Nowadays automated devices have developed for higher safety and efficacy. The devices have evolved to include corded and battery-powered pens (Figure 5.2), simultaneous vacuum and drug application, and needling rollers connected to a bottle from which a drug or active solution can be pushed into the skin while needling (Figure 5.3). These automated devices (Figure 5.4) offer more variation in number of needles, needle length, and speed, which allows operators to choose the appropriate needle and speed for each treatment.

Needle depth (0.25–3.0 mm) and speed can be customized to the pathology and treatment purpose. The sterilized cartridges are disposable, and contain between 6 and 36 needles, depending on the device [74]. Most needles' diameter is 30–33 gauge. The needles oscillate rapidly at either fixed or adjustable frequency. The specially designed tip is small (often 5–12 mm in diameter) and therefore it's easy to treat the narrow curves and contours on each part of the face. Some devices also have a tilting needle plate which allows even easier access to difficult areas with low epidermal trauma. This special design helps the tip to adapt to any surface of the skin and assure perpendicular needle penetration. It offers gentle but steady velocity of automated movements which more effectively and reliably penetrate

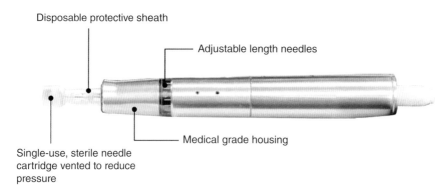

Disposable protective sheath

Adjustable length needles

Medical grade housing

Single-use, sterile needle
cartridge vented to reduce
pressure

Figure 5.2 Automated microneedling pens. *Source:* CANDELA CORPORATION. https://candelamedical.com/na/provider/product/exceed-microneedling.

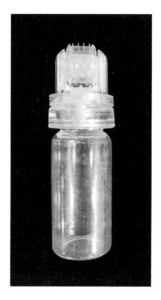

Figure 5.3 Needling roller (hydroroller) with a bottle connection to combine substance delivery during needling. *Source:* Atchima Suwanchinda.

the epidermis into the deep dermis, producing favorable results. The discomfort is much less at higher speeds versus lower speeds. There is less risk for needle stick or needles retracting when the needles are off the skin. With proper technique, it minimizes the risk of skin maceration or shearing. The sterility is ensured by single-use disposable cartridges. In addition, some devices have a special design of the safety membrane to prevent backflow of liquid, eliminating risk of contamination of the handpiece. Therefore, it is very important to choose only FDA-approved devices for MN treatment for reliable, safe, persistent, and effective results.

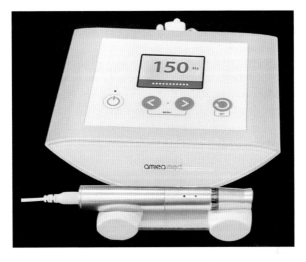

Figure 5.4 Automated microneedling device. *Source:* Atchima Suwanchinda.

Clinical considerations

- The devices are chosen according to operator preferences. Regardless of device, the MN treatment principles are similar and involve running needles vertically, horizontally, and diagonally under even pressure. Multiple passes should be done to ensure adequate surface coverage.
- The treatment plan should be justified according to anatomical location and clinical conditions. There is variation in tissue thickness and skin texture. At different locations the depth to penetrate papillary and/or reticular dermis requires different length needles. Cadaveric studies have shown facial skin thickness varies from approximately 0.5 mm depth at the upper eyelid to 1.6–1.9 mm at the lower nasal sidewall and upper lip. The neck may range 0.75–1.5 mm [104].
- There is no well-established, evidence-based MN treatment protocol for hyperpigmentation. There are use cases for both MN monotherapy and MN with combination drug delivery and laser treatment. Published studies have used needles of both 0.5mm and 1.5 mm length. Results from both depths showed statistically clinical improvement in pigmentation. The interval of treatment was also varied from two weeks and four weeks interval. The combination regimen used in various studies includes from cosmeceuticals, medical drugs, and bioactive agents, with various clinical response and side effects [8, 11, 59–61, 94].

Preprocedure care

The skin should be prepared with vitamin A and vitamin C formulations preoperatively for at least a month to maximize dermal collagen formation [2]. Vitamin A expresses its influence on 400–1,000 genes that are essential for proliferation and differentiation of all major cells in the epidermis and dermis [105–107]. Prolonged sun exposure should be avoided for at least 24 hours preprocedure to minimize excessive injury and inflammation. Any patient with active infection or sunburn at the treated area should resolve these conditions before MN treatment.

Before the microneedle procedure is performed, the treated area should be cleaned to remove any makeup or debris prior to anesthetization with topical anesthesia for 45–60 minutes [2, 108]. Alster et al. suggested that 30% lidocaine cream should be applied about 20–30 minutes before treatment [16].

Operative technique

- Remove the lidocaine cream with NSS-soaked gauze and prep the treated site with preferred antiseptics, alcohol, or chlorhexidine in alcohol or in water immediately before the procedure.
- Wait until the antiseptics dry before starting the procedure.
- Topical drugs or bioactive agents are typically applied to the treatment areas in order to facilitate gliding of the devices across the skin to prevent unseemly injury to the overlying epidermis (Figure 5.5).
- Additional agents can be added during the needling (Figure 5.6).
- Gentle skin traction is done while applying the MN tip perpendicular to the surface to create the smooth delivery of microneedles into the dermis.
- Firmly hold the device and move across the skin in circular motions over the treatment area or in a multidirectional or cross-hatching pattern until effacement of the lesion is seen or until pinpoint bleeding is observed (Figure 5.7).
- Several passes can be done to ensure the homogeneity of the treatment.
- Sterile, cold, NSS-soaked gauze is used to remove excess blood and achieve hemostasis. It also helps to ease skin comfort.
- A thin layer of healing-aid ointment, topical hydrocortisone-containing balm, or growth factor is immediately applied, according to preferences.

Postprocedure care

MN is generally well tolerated by patients and most patients can return to daily work the next day. Immediate after the treatment, the treated area is usually swollen, with

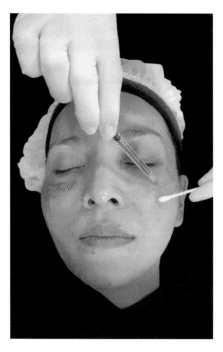

Figure 5.5 Topical agents of drugs or bioactive agents are typically applied to the treatment areas before needling treatment in order to facilitate gliding of the devices across the skin to prevent unseemly injury to the overlying epidermis. *Source:* Anchalee Srinakorn.

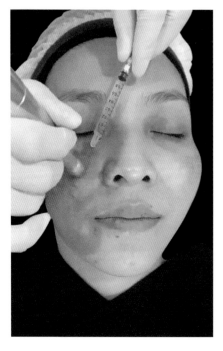

Figure 5.6 Topical agents of drugs or bioactive agents are added during the needling treatment. *Source:* Anchalee Srinakorn.

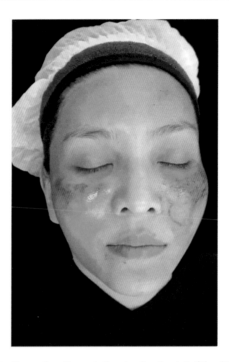

Figure 5.7 Pinpoint bleeding and erythema is the visual end point of the skin needling treatments. *Source:* Anchalee Srinakorn.

superficial bruising and bleeding which stops within a few hours. Serous ooze might be seen in some patients, which usually stops after few hours [5]. Patients may have a transient sunburnlike feeling for two to three hours, which can be treated with analgesics or hyaluronic acid–based hydrating serum [108]. Erythema usually subsides after 24 hours, with some areas of pinpoint bleeding that might become darker (Figure 5.8). Erythema and mild desquamation may be seen for about two to three days, or in some patients may last up to five days [5]. Mild edema can occur and may persist for two to three days after treatment. Antiviral drugs are indicated to prevent herpes simplex outbreaks in patients with history of previous HSV infection [108].

Home care is gentle cleansing with mild nonallergic cleanser followed by application of nonallergic healing-aid ointment or growth factor–containing gel several times a day. Local antibiotic creams may be prescribed [1]. It is important to avoid nonapproved substances for intradermal use due to higher risk of developing dermatitis and granuloma formation; the microchannels created by microneedle have been reported to remain open for several hours after treatment [109].

Sun avoidance should be strongly advised. The regular use of sunscreen with at least SPF 30 along with other sun-protective measures are advised as a routine [1]. Mineral (nonchemical) physical sunblock is recommended to avoid risk of post-treatment dyspigmentation. Makeup is to be avoided in the first 48 hours

(a)   (b)   (c)

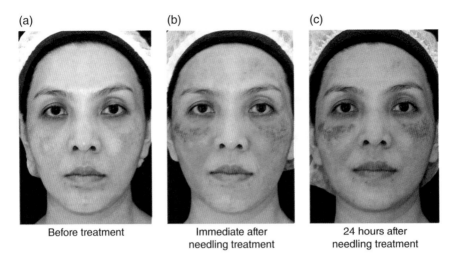

| Before treatment | Immediate after needling treatment | 24 hours after needling treatment |

Figure 5.8 (a) Before treatment. (b) Skin needling treatment on melasma patient showed erythema with pinpoint bleeding after 3 passes, which demonstrated the visual end point of the skin needling treatments. (c) After 24 hour the degree of Erythema subsided. Area of pinpoint bleeding became dark red. Mild desquamation was seen. *Source:* Anchalee Srinakorn.

post-treatment. Regular skincare and make up can be introduced after at least seven days, depending on the return of normal skin barrier or when erythema has resolved.

Additional treatment sessions are usually recommended, with at least a four-week interval (or, less commonly, a two-week interval) until the desired outcome is achieved. A maintenance session is also recommended after six months or one year to enhance the results [110].

Contraindications

Physicians should be aware of the contraindications to treatment with MN.

- Active pustular or cystic acne should be prescribed oral antibiotics to control outbreaks before performing the procedure – except when doing fractional MN radiofrequency which directly targets sebaceous glands, causing reduction in sebum production and hyperproliferation of keratinocytes [2].
- Patients with rosacea, fragile capillaries, or vascular lesions should not receive these procedures because telangiectasia and erythema maybe temporarily or permanently worsened [111].
- Individuals who have an active inflammation such as eczema, psoriasis, or lupus erythematosus, or a local infection such as herpes labialis or molluscum contagiosum within the treatment area should not be treated with MN [6].

- Patients who are currently on immunosuppressive drugs, chemo/radiotherapy, or anticoagulant therapy or who have blood dyscrasia should be excluded [2].
- Patients who have a tendency for hypertrophic scars or keloids are poor candidates [2].

Side effects and their management

Even though MN is a simple and minimally invasive procedure, complications can occur as a direct result of the procedure itself or from other combination modalities, particularly with transdermal drug delivery.

- **Postprocedural erythema** is the most common adverse effect, and its degree probably depends on various factors, including the site of MN application, the number of passes of MN application, MN needle length and device type, variability between skin types and combination treatment with topical products [112].
- **Contact dermatitis** from the concomitant use of MN with topical agents can occur, particularly allergic and irritant dermatitis. It is essential to note that there is a higher risk of these adverse effects if using non–FDA approved products for intradermal application [112]. Contact dermatitis as a result of arnica cream used after MN treatment was reported. But the patient applied topical arnica cream to the normal intact skin without further adverse effect [113]. The lesion had healed completely within 72 hours after topical corticosteroids application. Therefore, patients must be instructed on proper postprocedural care, particularly skincare product application for the first 24 hours, to avoid contact dermatitis and other adverse events. Only approved intradermal products should be applied after alteration of the skin barrier from MN treatment. This incident can increase the risk of hyperpigmentation, particularly in patients of color.
- **Lymphadenopathy** was previously reported in a patient who underwent MN with 0.5 mm and 1 mm–length needles on the face. A painful retroauricular lymph node developed on both sides of the face on the following day. It may be due to the tiny microtunneling generated by microneedles, where the normal flora bacteria could penetrate and probably stimulate inflammation and infection. A short course of oral antibiotic was prescribed to alleviate and shorten this adverse event [114].
- **Allergic granulomatous reaction** and systemic hypersensitivity associated with MN was reported in three patients studied by Soltani-Arabshahi et al. The substances used in this case were a high dose of lipophilic vitamin C (Vita C Serum™; Sanitas Skincare) and a gel product (Boske Hydra-Boost Gel™; Boske Dermaceuticals). The cutaneous symptoms presented with erythematous rash to the progressive well-demarcated erythematous indurated plaques with minimal overlying scale, and progressive facial indurated erythematous papules coalescing into plaques, swelling, and erythema nodosum. The symptoms can

occur several days to two weeks after treatment. Other systemic symptoms found were arthralgia at the knees, high fever, and fatigue. A biopsy of this abnormal skin reaction showed foreign body–type granulomatous reactions with focal, polarizable material detected in a few giant cells' cytoplasm. The tissue cultures for bacteria, mycobacteria, and fungus were negative. The patch testing of two patients showed a 1+ reaction to Vita C Serum at the 96-hour reading while prick testing for contact urticaria was negative. Topical corticosteroids alternating with topical calcineurin inhibitor failed to trigger a response. Gradual partial improvement was demonstrated with midpotency corticosteroid, a tapering dose of oral methylprednisolone, doxycycline 100 mg/d, or minocycline 100 mg/day for five days [115].

A similar incident was reported by Eisert et al. in a 57-year-old female patient who developed warm erythematous papules, some of which has coalesced to plaques two months after MN procedures at her lateral thighs. The histopathological findings were consistent with granuloma dermatitis with extensive, dense infiltration in the superficial, mid and deep dermis consisting of large histiocytes. The CD68 antibodies were strongly positive. Patch testing showed no evidence of hypersensitivity. Various treatments, including topical corticosteroid, tacrolimus, and systemic prednisolone, were ineffective. Therefore, doxycycline 200 mg per day was given in addition to topical treatment with tacrolimus. A total of 2.5 months of the aforementioned regimen showed only a slightly improvement. According to the increasing use of fumaric acid esters (the approved drug for the treatment of psoriasis in Germany) to treat granulomatous disease with successful results, Fumaderm® (off-label) was prescribed, and gradually increased to three tablets per day. After 14 weeks, there was significant fading and flattening of the lesions. Thus, the dose was tapered to two tablets per day and was continually given for another two months, with nearly complete clearance of the lesions [20].

- **Nickel hypersensitivity** has also been reported in MN treatment with a dermaroller (Derma India®, Tamil Nadu, India) containing stainless steel, titanium-coated 1.5 mm needles. No topical serum or chemical was applied before, during, or after the procedure. The erythema and edema at the treated site slowly developed and became intense within 24 hours and remained the same for few days. The edema partially subsided and multiple tiny erythematous papules and few vesiculopustular lesions developed. Oral prednisolone 30 mg daily was given for five days, along with application of a low-potency topical corticosteroid. Patch testing was performed three months later with nickel sulfate and titanium. The test was negative for titanium testing, but at 48 hours vesiculopustular infiltration with intense erythema developed and expanded beyond the margin of the nickel chamber site. However, the reaction had partially subsided at 96 hours after testing. Even though the needle tips in the dermaroller were covered with titanium, the needles themselves were made entirely of stainless steel. The patient was exposed to nickel owing to a part of the needle other than the tip having entered the skin, leading to possible development of contact dermatitis related to nickel that leached out from the needles. After a short course of topical and systemic corticosteroids, the patient improved significantly [116].

• **Hyperpigmentation was reported by** Dogra et al. in MN treatment for acne scarring. A dermaroller with 192 fine microneedles of 1.5 mm length and 0.1 mm diameter was used to treat 36 Asian patients with acne scars, in five monthly sessions. Postinflammatory hyperpigmentation was found in five patients. Three patients had particular severe hyperpigmentation; thus, they were dropped from the study. Two patients had only mild hyperpigmentation that ameliorated gradually after strict compliance with photoprotection guidelines [117]. However, compared to other skin resurfacing modalities, such as dermabrasion, chemical peels, and laser treatment, MN is considered to have a lower risk of hyperpigmentation [3]. In addition, the Dogra et al. study trial demonstrated that two patients had developed tram-track sign adverse effects. One patient had very severe tram-track scarring over the malar prominence area and was forced to withdraw from the trial. The lesion improved after topical tretinoin application. Another patient had less severe tram-track scarring and was able to complete the protocol. It was postulated that tram-track scarring may result from excessive force during the MN procedure over the bony prominence area of the face [117]. Even though MN therapy offers a lower risk of dyspigmentation than other treatment modalities, results depend on techniques, concomitant agents used, proper postoperative care, patient's skin condition, and other factors.

Summary

MN seems to be an effective modality for pigmentation problems, especially in patients of color. MN can be used alone or as a drug-delivery mechanism for depigmenting agents, PRP, or other biological substances. Even though there are no available evidence-base treatment protocols, MN auspiciously gives favorable results for the treatment of hyperpigmentation disorders.

References

1 Doddaballapur S. Microneedling with dermaroller. J Cutan Aesthet Surg. 2009;2(2): 110–111.

2 Singh A, Yadav S. Microneedling: advances and widening horizons. Indian Dermatol Online J. 2016;7(4):244–254.

3 Cohen BE, Elbuluk N. Microneedling in skin of color: a review of uses and efficacy. J Am Acad Dermatol. 2016;74(2):348–355.

4 Bonati LM, Epstein GK, Strugar TL. Microneedling in all skin types: a review. J Drugs Dermatol. 2017;16(4):308–313.

5 Aust MC, Fernandes D, Kolokythas P, et al. Percutaneous collagen induction therapy: an alternative treatment for scars, wrinkles, and skin laxity. Plast Reconstr Surg. 2008;121(4):1421–1429.

6 Hou A, Cohen B, Haimovic A, Elbuluk N. Microneedling: a comprehensive review. Dermatol Surg. 2017;43(3):321–339.

7 Konicke K, Knabel M, Olasz E. Microneedling in dermatology: a review. Plast Surg Nurs. 2017;37(3):112–115.

8 Sahni K, Kassir M. DermaFracTM: an innovative new treatment for periorbital melanosis in a dark-skinned male patient. J Cutan Aesthet Surg. 2013;6(3):158–160.

9 Lima EA. Microneedling in facial recalcitrant melasma: report of a series of 22 cases. An Bras Dermatol. 2015;90(6):919–921.

10 Lima EVA, Lima M, Paixao MP, Miot HA. Assessment of the effects of skin microneedling as adjuvant therapy for facial melasma: a pilot study. BMC Dermatol. 2017;17(1):14.

11 Cassiano DP, Esposito ACC, Hassun KM, et al. Early clinical and histological changes induced by microneedling in facial melasma: a pilot study. Indian J Dermatol Venereol Leprol. 2019;85(6):638–641.

12 Ustuner P, Balevi A, Ozdemir M. A split-face, investigator-blinded comparative study on the efficacy and safety of Q-switched Nd:YAG laser plus microneedling with vitamin C versus Q-switched Nd:YAG laser for the treatment of recalcitrant melasma. J Cosmet Laser Ther. 2017;19(7):383–390.

13 Mikszta JA, Alarcon JB, Brittingham JM, et al. Improved genetic immunization via micromechanical disruption of skin-barrier function and targeted epidermal delivery. Nat Med. 2002;8(4):415–419.

14 Donnelly RF, Morrow DIJ, McCarron PA, et al. Microneedle-mediated intradermal delivery of 5-aminolevulinic acid: potential for enhanced topical photodynamic therapy. Journal of Controlled Release. 2008;129(3):154–162.

15 Mukerjee EV, Collins SD, Isseroff RR, Smith RL. Microneedle array for transdermal biological fluid extraction and in situ analysis. Sensors and Actuators A: Physical. 2004;114(2):267–275.

16 Alster TS, Graham PM. Microneedling: a review and practical guide. Dermatol Surg. 2018;44(3):397–404.

17 Hashim PW, Levy Z, Cohen JL, Goldenberg G. Microneedling therapy with and without platelet-rich plasma. Cutis. 2017;99(4):239–242.

18 Aust MC, Reimers K, Kaplan HM, et al. Percutaneous collagen induction-regeneration in place of cicatrisation? J Plast Reconstr Aesthet Surg. 2011;64(1):97–107.

19 Aust MC, Reimers K, Gohritz A, et al. Percutaneous collagen induction. Scarless skin rejuvenation: fact or fiction? Clin Exp Dermatol. 2010;35(4):437–439.

20 Eisert L, Zidane M, Waigandt I, et al. Granulomatous reaction following microneedling of striae distensae. J Dtsch Dermatol Ges. 2019;17(4):443–445.

21 Liebl H, Kloth LC. Skin cell proliferation stimulated by microneedles. The Journal of the American College of Clinical Wound Specialists. 2012;4(1):2–6.

22 Fernandes D. Minimally invasive percutaneous collagen induction. Oral Maxillofac Surg Clin North Am. 2005;17(1):51–63, vi.

23　Vandervoort J, Ludwig A. Microneedles for transdermal drug delivery: a minireview. Front Biosci. 2008;13:1711–1715.

24　Ramaut L, Hoeksema H, Pirayesh A, et al. Microneedling:where do we stand now? A systematic review of the literature. J Plast Reconstr Aesthet Surg. 2018;71(1):1–14.

25　Cichorek M, Wachulska M, Stasiewicz A, Tyminska A. Skin melanocytes: biology and development. Postepy Dermatol Alergol. 2013;30(1):30–41.

26　Moustakas A. TGF-beta targets PAX3 to control melanocyte differentiation. Dev Cell. 2008;15(6):797–799.

27　Hirobe T. Keratinocytes regulate the function of melanocytes. Dermatologica Sinica. 2014;32(4):200–204.

28　Iriarte C, Awosika O, Rengifo-Pardo M, Ehrlich A. Review of applications of microneedling in dermatology. Clinical, Cosmetic and Investigational Dermatology. 2017;10:289–298.

29　Rajanala S, Maymone MBC, Vashi NA. Melasma pathogenesis: a review of the latest research, pathological findings, and investigational therapies. Dermatol Online J. 2019;25(10).

30　Sarkar R, Bansal A, Ailawadi P. Future therapies in melasma: what lies ahead? Indian J Dermatol Venereol Leprol. 2020;86(1):8–17.

31　Kwon SH, Na JI, Choi JY, Park KC. Melasma: updates and perspectives. Exp Dermatol. 2019;28(6):704–708.

32　Passeron T, Picardo M. Melasma, a photoaging disorder. Pigment Cell Melanoma Res. 2018;31(4):461–465.

33　Lee BW, Schwartz RA, Janniger CK. Melasma. G Ital Dermatol Venereol. 2017;152(1):36–45.

34　Handel AC, Miot LD, Miot HA. Melasma: a clinical and epidemiological review. An Bras Dermatol. 2014;89(5):771–782.

35　Torres-Alvarez B, Mesa-Garza IG, Castanedo-Cazares JP, et al. Histochemical and immunohistochemical study in melasma: evidence of damage in the basal membrane. Am J Dermatopathol. 2011;33(3):291–295.

36　Esposito ACC, Brianezi G, de Souza NP, et al. Ultrastructural characterization of damage in the basement membrane of facial melasma. Arch Dermatol Res. 2019.

37　Kwon SH, Hwang YJ, Lee SK, Park KC. Heterogeneous Pathology of Melasma and Its Clinical Implications. Int J Mol Sci. 2016;17(6).

38　Hernandez-Barrera R, Torres-Alvarez B, Castanedo-Cazares JP, et al. Solar elastosis and presence of mast cells as key features in the pathogenesis of melasma. Clin Exp Dermatol. 2008;33(3):305–308.

39　Kang WH, Yoon KH, Lee ES, et al. Melasma: histopathological characteristics in 56 Korean patients. Br J Dermatol. 2002;146(2):228–237.

40　Kim EH, Kim YC, Lee ES, Kang HY. The vascular characteristics of melasma. J Dermatol Sci. 2007;46(2):111–116.

41　Ogbechie-Godec OA, Elbuluk N. Melasma: an up-to-date comprehensive review. Dermatol Ther (Heidelb). 2017;7(3):305–318.

42　Gupta AK, Gover MD, Nouri K, Taylor S. The treatment of melasma: a review of clinical trials. J Am Acad Dermatol. 2006;55(6):1048–1065.

43　Murthy R, Roos JCP, Goldberg RA. Periocular hyaluronic acid fillers: applications, implications, complications. Curr Opin Ophthalmol. 2019;30(5):395–400.

44 van Smeden J, Janssens M, Boiten WA, et al. Intercellular skin barrier lipid composition and organization in Netherton syndrome patients. J Invest Dermatol. 2014;134(5):1238–1245.

45 Trommer H, Neubert RH. Overcoming the stratum corneum: the modulation of skin penetration. A review. Skin Pharmacol Physiol. 2006;19(2):106–121.

46 Hadgraft J. Skin, the final frontier. Int J Pharm. 2001;224(1–2):1–18.

47 Santoianni P, Nino M, Calabro G. Intradermal drug delivery by low-frequency sonophoresis (25 kHz). Dermatol Online J. 2004;10(2):24.

48 Rastogi SK, Singh J. Effect of chemical penetration enhancer and iontophoresis on the in vitro percutaneous absorption enhancement of insulin through porcine epidermis. Pharm Dev Technol. 2005;10(1):97–104.

49 Denet AR, Vanbever R, Preat V. Skin electroporation for transdermal and topical delivery. Adv Drug Deliv Rev. 2004;56(5):659–674.

50 Hui SW. Overview of drug delivery and alternative methods to electroporation. Methods Mol Biol. 2008;423:91–107.

51 Telang PS. Vitamin C in dermatology. Indian Dermatol Online J. 2013;4(2):143–146.

52 Wu S, Shi H, Wu H, et al. Treatment of melasma with oral administration of tranexamic acid. Aesthetic Plast Surg. 2012;36(4):964–970.

53 Dunn CJ, Goa KL. Tranexamic Acid. Drugs. 1999;57(6):1005–1032.

54 Taraz M, Niknam S, Ehsani AH. Tranexamic acid in treatment of melasma: a comprehensive review of clinical studies. Dermatol Ther. 2017;30(3).

55 Kim SJ, Park JY, Shibata T, et al. Efficacy and possible mechanisms of topical tranexamic acid in melasma. Clin Exp Dermatol. 2016;41(5):480–485.

56 Lee JH, Park JG, Lim SH, et al. Localized intradermal microinjection of tranexamic acid for treatment of melasma in Asian patients: a preliminary clinical trial. Dermatol Surg. 2006;32(5):626–631.

57 Tan AWM, Sen P, Chua SH, Goh BK. Oral tranexamic acid lightens refractory melasma. Australas J Dermatol. 2017;58(3):e105-e108.

58 Perper M, Eber AE, Fayne R, et al. Tranexamic acid in the treatment of melasma: a review of the literature. Am J Clin Dermatol. 2017;18(3):373–381.

59 Ismail ESA, Patsatsi A, Abd El-Maged WM, Nada E. Efficacy of microneedling with topical vitamin C in the treatment of melasma. J Cosmet Dermatol. 2019.

60 Fabbrocini G, De Vita V, Fardella N, et al. Skin needling to enhance depigmenting serum penetration in the treatment of melasma. Plast Surg Int. 2011;2011:158241.

61 Budamakuntla L, Loganathan E, Suresh DH, et al. A randomised, open-label, comparative study of tranexamic acid microinjections and tranexamic acid with microneedling in patients with melasma. J Cutan Aesthet Surg. 2013;6(3):139–143.

62 Badran MM, Kuntsche J, Fahr A. Skin penetration enhancement by a microneedle device (Dermaroller) in vitro: dependency on needle size and applied formulation. Eur J Pharm Sci. 2009;36(4–5):511–523.

63 Sarkar R. Idiopathic cutaneous hyperchromia at the orbital region or periorbital hyperpigmentation. J Cutan Aesthet Surg. 2012;5(3):183–184.

64 Roberts WE. Periorbital hyperpigmentation: review of etiology, medical evaluation, and aesthetic treatment. J Drugs Dermatol. 2014;13(4):472–482.

65 Sheth PB, Shah HA, Dave JN. Periorbital hyperpigmentation: a study of its prevalence, common causative factors and its association with personal habits and other disorders. Indian J Dermatol. 2014;59(2):151–157.

66 Kontochristopoulos G, Kouris A, Platsidaki E, et al. Combination of microneedling and 10% trichloroacetic acid peels in the management of infraorbital dark circles. J Cosmet Laser Ther. 2016;18(5):289–292.

67 Mitsuishi T, Shimoda T, Mitsui Y, et al. The effects of topical application of phytonadione, retinol and vitamins C and E on infraorbital dark circles and wrinkles of the lower eyelids. J Cosmet Dermatol. 2004;3(2):73–75.

68 Epstein JS. Management of infraorbital dark circles. A significant cosmetic concern. Arch Facial Plast Surg. 1999;1(4):303–307.

69 Ma G, Lin XX, Hu XJ, et al. Treatment of venous infraorbital dark circles using a long-pulsed 1,064-nm neodymium-doped yttrium aluminum garnet laser. Dermatol Surg. 2012;38(8):1277–1282.

70 Roh MR, Kim TK, Chung KY. Treatment of infraorbital dark circles by autologous fat transplantation: a pilot study. Br J Dermatol. 2009;160(5):1022–1025.

71 Sahni K, Kassir M. Dermafrac: an innovative new treatment for periorbital melanosis in a dark-skinned male patient. J Cutan Aesthet Surg. 2013;6(3):158–160.

72 Kubiak M, Mucha P, Debowska R, Rotsztejn H. Evaluation of 70% glycolic peels versus 15% trichloroacetic peels for the treatment of photodamaged facial skin in aging women. Dermatol Surg. 2014;40(8):883–891.

73 Wang N, Liu H, Li X, et al. Activities of MSCs derived from transgenic mice seeded on ADM scaffolds in wound healing and assessment by advanced optical techniques. Cell Physiol Biochem. 2017;42(2):623–639.

74 Duncan DI. Microneedling with biologicals: advantages and limitations. Facial Plast Surg Clin North Am. 2018;26(4):447–454.

75 Haak C, Hannibal J, Paasch U, et al. Laser-induced thermal coagulation enhances skin uptake of topically applied compounds. Lasers Surg Med. 2017;49(6):582–591.

76 Kalluri H, Kolli CS, Banga AK. Characterization of microchannels created by metal microneedles: formation and closure. AAPS J. 2011;13(3):473–481.

77 Olesen UH, Mogensen M, Haedersdal M. Vehicle type affects filling of fractional laser-ablated channels imaged by optical coherence tomography. Lasers Med Sci. 2017;32(3):679–684.

78 Li ZJ, Choi HI, Choi DK, et al. Autologous platelet-rich plasma: a potential therapeutic tool for promoting hair growth. Dermatol Surg. 2012;38(7pt1):1040–1046.

79 Marx REJId. Platelet-rich plasma (PRP): what is PRP and what is not PRP? Implant Dent. 2001;10(4):225–228.

80 Kon E, Filardo G, Di Martino A, Marcacci M. Platelet-rich plasma (PRP) to treat sports injuries: evidence to support its use. Knee Surg Sports Traumatol Arthrosc. 2011;19(4):516–527.

81 Hausauer AK, Jones DH. PRP and Microneedling in Aesthetic Medicine: Thieme; 2019.

82 Çayırlı M, Çalışkan E, Açıkgöz G, et al. Regression of melasma with platelet-rich plasma treatment. Ann Dermatol. 2014;26(3):401–402.

83 Amini F, Ramasamy T, Yew CH. Response to intradermal autologous platelet rich plasma injection in refractory dermal melasma: Report of two cases. JUMMEC. 2015;18(2):1–6.

84 Hofny ER, Abdel-Motaleb AA, Ghazally A, et al. Platelet-rich plasma is a useful therapeutic option in melasma. J Dermatolog Treat. 2019;30(4):396–401.

85 Sirithanabadeekul P, Dannarongchai A, Suwanchinda A. Platelet-rich plasma treatment for melasma: A pilot study. J Cosmet Dermatol. 2019.

86 Lapeere H, Boone B, Schepper S, et al. Hypomelanoses and hypermelanoses. 2008;7: 622–640.

87 De La Mata J. Platelet rich plasma. A new treatment tool for the rheumatologist? Reumatol Clin. 2013;9(3):166–171.

88 Kim DS, Park SH, Park KC. Transforming growth factor-β1 decreases melanin synthesis via delayed extracellular signal-regulated kinase activation. Int J Biochem Cell Biol. 2004;36(8):1482–1491.

89 Yang G, Li Y, Nishimura EK, et al. Inhibition of PAX3 by TGF-β modulates melanocyte viability. Mol Cell. 2008;32(4):554–563.

90 Yun WJ, Bang SH, Min KH, et al. Epidermal growth factor and epidermal growth factor signaling attenuate laser-induced melanogenesis. Dermatol Surg. 2013;39(12): 1903–1911.

91 Moubasher AE, Youssef EM, Abou-Taleb DAE. Q-switched Nd: YAG laser versus trichloroacetic acid peeling in the treatment of melasma among Egyptian patients. Dermatol Surg. 2014;40(8):874–882.

92 Mochtar M, Ilona SE, Zulfikar D, et al. A split-face of dermaroller and intradermal injection with the autologous platelet rich fibrin lysate in the treatment of exogenous ocronosis: A case series. 2019.

93 Cha J, Falanga V. Stem cells in cutaneous wound healing. Clin Dermatol. 2007;25(1):73–78.

94 Lee HJ, Lee EG, Kang S, et al. Efficacy of microneedling plus human stem cell conditioned medium for skin rejuvenation: a randomized, controlled, blinded split-face study. Ann Dermatol. 2014;26(5):584–591.

95 Kim WS, Park SH, Ahn SJ, et al. Whitening effect of adipose-derived stem cells: a critical role of TGF-β1. Biol Pharm Bull. 2008;31(4):606–610.

96 Javelaud D, Alexaki VI, Mauviel A. Transforming growth factor-β in cutaneous melanoma. Pigment Cell Melanoma Res. 2008;21(2):123–132.

97 Jeon BJ, Kim DW, Kim MS, et al. Protective effects of adipose-derived stem cells against UVB-induced skin pigmentation. J Plast Surg Hand Surg. 2016;50(6): 336–342.

98 Klar AS, Biedermann T, Michalak K, et al. Human adipose mesenchymal cells inhibit melanocyte differentiation and the pigmentation of human skin via increased expression of TGF-β1. J Investig Dermatol. 2017;137(12):2560–2569.

99 Nishimura EK, Suzuki M, Igras V, et al. Key roles for transforming growth factor β in melanocyte stem cell maintenance. Cell Stem Cell. 2010;6(2):130–140.

100 Kim WS, Park BS, Sung JH. Protective role of adipose-derived stem cells and their soluble factors in photoaging. Arch Dermatol Res. 2009;301(5):329–336.

101 Lee MJ, Kim J, Lee KI, et al. Enhancement of wound healing by secretory factors of endothelial precursor cells derived from human embryonic stem cells. Cytotherapy. 2011;13(2):165–178.

102 Fitzpatrick RE, Rostan EF. Reversal of photodamage with topical growth factors: a pilot study. J Cosmet Laser Ther. 2003;5(1):25–34.

103 Bos JD, Meinardi M. The 500 Dalton rule for the skin penetration of chemical compounds and drugs. Exp Dermatol. 2000;9(3):165–169.

104 Chopra K, Calva D, Sosin M, et al. A comprehensive examination of topographic thickness of skin in the human face. Aesthet Surg J. 2015;35(8):1007–13.

105 Bernard FX, Pedretti N, Rosdy M, Deguercy A. Comparison of gene expression profiles in human keratinocyte mono-layer cultures, reconstituted epidermis and normal human skin; transcriptional effects of retinoid treatments in reconstituted human epidermis. Exp Dermatol. 2002;11(1):59–74.

106 Rosdahl I, Andersson E, Kagedal B, Torma H. Vitamin A metabolism and mRNA expression of retinoid-binding protein and receptor genes in human epidermal melanocytes and melanoma cells. Melanoma Res. 1997;7(4):267–274.

107 Johnstone CC, Farley A. The physiological basics of wound healing. Nurs Stand. 2005;19(43):59–65; quiz 6.

108 Lee JC, Daniels MA, Roth MZ. Mesotherapy, microneedling, and chemical peels. Clin Plast Surg. 2016;43(3):583–595.

109 Bal S, Kruithof A, Liebl H, et al. In vivo visualization of microneedle conduits in human skin using laser scanning microscopy. Laser Physics Letters. 2010;7(3):242–246.

110 El-Domyati M, Barakat M, Awad S, et al. Multiple microneedling sessions for minimally invasive facial rejuvenation: an objective assessment. Int J Dermatol. 2015;54(12):1361–1369.

111 Bhalla M, Thami GP. Microdermabrasion: reappraisal and brief review of literature. Dermatol Surg. 2006;32(6):809–814.

112 Cary JH, Li BS, Maibach HI. Dermatotoxicology of microneedles (MNs) in man. Biomed Microdevices. 2019;21(3):66.

113 Cercal Fucci-da-Costa AP, Reich Camasmie H. Drug delivery after microneedling: report of an adverse reaction. Dermatol Surg. 2018;44(4):593–594.

114 Elghblawi E. Intense retroauricular lymphadenopathy post-microneedling. J Cosmet Dermatol. 2019;18(6):2048–2049.

115 Soltani-Arabshahi R, Wong JW, Duffy KL, Powell DL. Facial allergic granulomatous reaction and systemic hypersensitivity associated with microneedle therapy for skin rejuvenation. JAMA Dermatol. 2014;150(1):68–72.

116 Yadav S, Dogra S. A cutaneous reaction to microneedling for postacne scarring caused by nickel hypersensitivity. Aesthet Surg J. 2016;36(4):NP168–170.

117 Dogra S, Yadav S, Sarangal R. Microneedling for acne scars in Asian skin type: an effective low cost treatment modality. J Cosmet Dermatol. 2014;13(3):180–187.

6

Treatment of Acne and Acne Scars with Microneedling

Stuti Khare Shukla[1] and Michael H. Gold[2]

[1]Elements of Aesthetics Clinics, Dr. Stuti Khare's Skin & Hair Clinics, Mumbai, India
[2]Gold Skin Care Center, Tennessee Clinical Research Center, Nashville, TN, USA

Background

Acne and its prevalence

Acne vulgaris is a chronic inflammatory condition of the pilosebaceous unit [1, 2]. It can be seen as open or closed comedones or both, and as inflammatory lesions – including papules, pustules, or nodules [3]. Acne vulgaris is among the top 10 most prevalent conditions worldwide and it is one of the most common skin conditions [4]. Some degree of acne affects almost all adolescents between 15 and 17 years of age [5, 2]. Up to 80% of adolescents and up to 5% of adults experience acne [6]. The impact of acne on quality of life can be profound [7].

Compared to people without acne, individuals with acne are at a higher risk of experiencing depression and anxiety, especially in those whose quality of life has been affected [8]. They are more likely to have lower self-esteem and lower body satisfaction [9]. Optimal treatments may significantly improve the appearance, quality of life, and self-esteem of affected people [9].

Etiology of acne and pathogenesis of acne scars

The pathogenesis of acne is currently attributed to multiple factors, such as increased sebum production, alteration of the quality of sebum lipids, androgen activity, proliferation of Propionibacterium acnes (P. acnes) within the follicle, and follicular hyperkeratinization [10].

Microneedling: Global Perspectives in Aesthetic Medicine, First Edition.
Edited by Elizabeth Bahar Houshmand.
© 2021 John Wiley & Sons Ltd. Published 2021 by John Wiley & Sons Ltd.

As sebum and keratinocytes hold together, the keratotic plug gradually forms and obstructs the pilosebaceous ducts, finally creating microcomedones [11]. In the past, colonization with Cutibacterium (formerly Propionibacterium) acnes (C. acnes) was thought to be the trigger of immune response in sebocytes, keratinocytes, and monocytes. However, recent investigations suggest that the dysbiosis targeting mainly C. acnes together with the activation of the innate immunity might lead to the chronic inflammatory response in acne vulgaris [12].

Pilosebaceous follicles in acne lesions are surrounded by macrophages expressing TLR2 on their surface. TLR2 activation leads to triggering of the transcription nuclear factor and the production of cytokines/chemokines [13]. All these events stimulate the infrainfundibular inflammatory process, follicular rupture, and perifollicular abscess formation, which stimulate the wound-healing process. Injury to the skin initiates a cascade of wound-healing events. Wound healing is one of the most complex biological processes and involves soluble chemical mediators and extracellular matrix components [13].

Pathogenesis of acne scars

The wound-healing process progresses through three stages: (i) inflammation, (ii) granulation tissue formation, and (iii) matrix remodeling [14, 15].

(i) Inflammation. This step plays an important role in the development of post-acne erythema and hyperpigmentation and the development of scarring, suggesting that treating early inflammation in acne lesions may be the best approach to revent acne scarring [16].

(ii) Granulation tissue formation. Damaged tissues are repaired and new capillaries are formed. Neutrophils are replaced by monocytes that change into macrophages and release several growth factors, including platelet-derived growth factor. New production of collagen by fibroblasts begins approximately three to five days after the wound is created [17].

(iii) Matrix remodeling. Fibroblasts and keratinocytes produce enzymes, including those that determine the architecture of the extracellular matrix metalloproteinases (MMPs) and tissue inhibitors of MMPs. MMPs are extracellular matrix (ECM)–degrading enzymes that interact and form a lytic cascade. As a consequence, an imbalance in the ratio of MMPs to tissue inhibitors of MMPs results in the development of atrophic or hypertrophic scars [18–20].

Epidemiology and types of acne scars

Scarring, as a physical disfigurement, is a frequent complication of acne. The psychological impact of scarring can be profound; scars can occur as a result of damage to the skin during the healing of active acne scarring [21]. Although active acne can persist for a decade or more, acne scars may persist for a lifetime [22]. One publication on the prevalence of acne scarring suggests that the type and extent of scarring correlates with the site and severity of previous acne and duration of acne before effective treatment. Facial scarring affects both sexes equally and occurs in up to 95% of cases scarring [23]. Several classifications and scales have been proposed for facial acne scarring [24]. Often, scarring is the consequence of severe inflammatory nodulocystic acne, but it may also be the product of superficial inflamed lesions or the squeezing or picking of lesions with the fingernails [21]. There are three general types of acne scars, depending on hyperproliferation or loss of collagen: hypertrophic scars, keloid scars, and atrophic scars. A person might have one or more types of scarring occurring in the same skin area [25, 26]. Inadequate healing response results in diminished deposition of collagen factors and formation of an atrophic scar, whereas if the healing response is too exuberant, a raised nodule of fibrotic tissue forms hypertrophic scars and keloids [27].

Of people with acne scars, 80–90% develop atrophic scars compared with a minority who develop hypertrophic scars. Atrophic scars can be further subclassified into ice pick, rolling, and boxcar [6]. The exact prevalence of each scar type is hard to calculate, but some estimations report that within atrophic scars, the ice pick type represents 60–70%, boxcar 20–30%, and rolling 15–25% [1, 6]. Each of these scar types has been classified based on the underlying scar pathology. Icepick scars are narrow (<2 mm) and extend vertically into the deep dermis or subcutaneous tissue [6]. Rolling scars have sloped and shallow borders with a normal skin texture at the base and are about 4–5 mm wide [6]. These scars result from abnormal fibrous bands anchoring the dermis to the subcutis, which produces a dell in the skin. Treatment is aimed at correcting the abnormal fibrous anchoring of these scars. Finally, boxcar scars are round to oval or rectangular depressions with sharply defined vertical edges that can be shallow (0.1–0.5 mm) or deep (>0.5). Shallow boxcar scars, rather than deep boxcar scars, are more amenable to treatment with resurfacing modalities [6].

Description of various interventions

Acne scars have always been challenging to treat. Different factors, e.g. color, texture, and morphology, can affect the treatment choice for each individual scar [25]. Early effective treatment of acne is probably the best strategy to prevent or limit postacne scarring [24, 2].

Many therapeutic approaches have been used to treat acne scarring, including both invasive and noninvasive methods. Unfortunately, even with the most expensive techniques it is difficult to achieve the goal of complete improvement. Thus, there is an ever-increasing demand for less invasive, highly effective treatments [28].

Microneedling therapy, or percutaneous collagen induction, is a new addition to the treatment modalities for such scars and has been reported to be simple and effective in atrophic acne scar treatment [29]. Other non-energy-based devices include subcision, (micro) dermabrasion, dermal fillers, and chemical peels.

Chemical peels can be helpful in treating mild acne lesions and shallow atrophic acne, which respond well to mild and medium-depth peels, such as 20–35% trichloroacetic acid (TCA), alpha hydroxy acids, salicylic acid, and Jessener's solution [6].

In the past decade, chemical reconstruction using TCA (CROSS) has come into favor for ice pick scars. In the CROSS method, high concentrations of TCA are applied on a sharp wooden applicator and then pressed firmly into the atrophic acne scars, and white frosting is observed [30]. The high concentrations of TCA cause coagulative necrosis of the epidermis, and the resultant wound healing causes an increase in the production of collagen and improvement in scar appearance [31]. However, these chemical peels have limited use for deeper atrophic scars, and should be used cautiously in darker-skinned patients because of the potential for pigmentary alterations. Deep chemical peels have fallen out of favor for the treatment of acne scars because of their significant side effect profile, such as dyschromia and scarring [32].

Punch excision is an excellent option for the treatment of icepick and deep boxcar scars. In this method, a punch biopsy instrument is used to remove deep atrophic scar tissue to the level of the subcutaneous fat and then closed with sutures [6]. It has been associated with good results, but secondary widening of the scar may occur.

Dermabrasion involves the use of sandpaper and hydrogen peroxide for hemostasis, or a rotating motorized handpiece attached to a serrated wheel, wire brush, or diamond-embedded fraises to remove the epidermis and upper dermis [33, 34].

By removing the superficial layers of the skin, the wound-healing process creates a smoother and more regular appearance of the scar, and new collagen is formed [6]. Dermabrasion is useful for superficial atrophic acne scars, such as rolling or shallow boxcar scars, but is less effective for icepick scars [31].

Injectable fillers used for atrophic scars have been proposed to improve the appearance of acne scars; collagen, autologous fat transfer, and artificial injectable fillers are most commonly used [35]. Their effect lasts 3–18 months, depending on the type of filler used. Hyaluronic acids (HA) are temporary fillers that last 3–12 months [6]. Hasson and Romero treated 12 patients with acne scars using HA (Esthélis, Anteis, S.A., Geneva, Switzerland); 74% had good to excellent results [36]. A 68% reduction in acne scars was seen in a recent study in five patients who had two treatments of HA with a modified vertical tower technique [2].

Among the energy-based devices, traditional ablative laser resurfacing have been used for treating acne scars. It removes the epidermis and part of the dermis of the scars, allowing collagen remodeling and re-epithelialization [21]. Patients typically do not need more than one treatment, but the treatment has adverse effects including persistent erythema, hypopigmentation, hyperpigmentation, infections, and scarring. It also has a very long recovery period (up to two weeks) [24].

Nonablative laser resurfacing produces dermal thermal injury while preserving the epidermis; this dermal thermal injury promotes collagen remodeling through the formation of new collagen, which leads to an improvement in scarring [37].

Fractional laser resurfacing acts, as the name indicates, "on regularly-spaced arrays over a fraction of the skin surface to induce thermal ablation of microscopic columns of epidermal and dermal tissue" [38]. This approach is more effective than nonablative resurfacing while providing a faster recovery than ablative resurfacing [39].

Problems related to aforementioned traditional energy-based devices prompted the development of nonablative methods, which owe their efficacy to triggering dermal neocollagenesis while preserving the stratum corneum and the epidermal barrier function. But the use of energy (in nonablative lasers, fractional lasers, and intense pulsed light lasers) for this purpose still entails problems with thermal injury and necrosis [40].

Microneedling treatment

Microneedling (MN), also known as collagen induction therapy, is a relatively new option for treatment of acne scars. The reported high efficacy, safety, and minimal post-treatment recovery rates associated with microneedling have increased its popularity among patients and clinicians [41].

The process involves repetitive puncturing of the skin with sterilized microneedles. Its original conception can be traced back to 1995, when Orentreich and Orentreich developed the concept of *subcision*, or using hypodermic needles to induce wound healing in depressed cutaneous scars. The process involved the insertion and maneuvering of a tribeveled hypodermic needle into the skin under the cutaneous defects to disrupt the underlying connective tissue that tethered down the skin in these area scars [41].

In 2006, Fernandes developed the first MN product, which became the modern-day Dermaroller® (Dermaroller Deutschland GmbH, Wolfenbuettel, Germany) [29].

The roller is a drum-shaped device with very fine protruding stainless steel needles (0.25–3mm in length) to delicately puncture the skin [42]. Research has been conducted in both animals and humans to elucidate the mechanism by which microneedling works. It has been hypothesized that the creation of numerous microchannels in atrophic acne scars physically breaks apart the compact collagen bundles in the superficial layer of the dermis while simultaneously inducing the production of new collagen and elastin underneath the scar [43, 44]. The creation of abundant microwounds directly stimulates the release of various growth factors that play a direct role in collagen and elastin synthesis and deposition within the dermis.

More specifically, the creation of microchannels induces a controlled skin injury with minimal epidermal damage and stimulates the dermal wound-healing cascade (inflammation, proliferation, and remodeling) to take place. This leads to the release of platelet-derived growth factor, fibroblast growth factor (FGF), and transforming growth factor alpha and beta (TGFα and TGFβ) [29, 45]. Neovascularization and neocollagenesis occur secondary to fibroblast proliferation and migration [46]. After the cutaneous injury, a fibronectin network is reated, providing a matrix for collagen type III deposition, which is eventually is replaced by type I collagen. This transition can occur over weeks to months [47]. The depth of neocollagenesis has been found to be 5–600 μm with a 1.5 mm length needle. Histological examination of the skin treated with four microneedling sessions one month apart showed up to 400% increase in collagen and elastin deposition at six months postoperatively, with a thickened stratum spinosum and normal rete ridges at one year postoperatively [47]. Collagen fiber bundles appear to have a normal lattice pattern rather than parallel bundles as in scar tissue [48]. Based on histologic analyses one year after a series of microneedling sessions, increased collagen deposition in the reticular dermis with a normal lattice architecture, increased elastic fiber deposition, a thickened epidermis (granular layer hyperplasia), and a normal stratum corneum and rete ridges have been shown [48]. Aust and colleagues demonstrated upregulation of TGFβ3, which promotes regeneration and scarless wound healing. The altered ratio after microneedling of TGFβ3 over TGFβ1 and TGFβ2 (the latter being responsible for fibrotic scarring) may partially explain the beneficial basis of this procedure [48].

Liebl and Kloth have proposed another hypothesis to explain how microneedling works [49]. The resting electrical membrane potential of cells is approximately −70 mV, and when needles come near the membrane, the inner electrical potential increases quickly to −100 mV. This triggers increased cell activity and the release of various proteins, potassium, and growth factors from the cells into the exterior, leading to the migration of fibroblasts to the site of injury, and hence collagen induction. Thus, the needles do not create a wound in a real sense, but rather body cells are fooled into believing that an injury has occurred [50–52]. However, more research needs to be done to elucidate the chain of events clearly.

Procedure

Microneedling is a simple office-based procedure performed under local anesthesia and lasting 10 to 20 minutes, depending on the area to be treated. The skin is stretched with one hand, and perpendicular rolling is done five times each in the horizontal, vertical, and oblique directions with the other hand [53]. The treatment endpoint is identified as uniform pinpoint bleeding which is easily controllable [53]. The procedure is well tolerated by patients and there are usually no post-treatment sequelae except slight erythema and edema lasting two to three days. There is no downtime and the patient can resume daily work the very next day. Treatments are performed at three-to-eight-week intervals and multiple sittings are needed to achieve the desired effect on the skin.

Various types of microneedling devices

Currently, there are many mechanical MN devices registered with the US Food and Drug Administration (FDA), with the majority being a variation of either the Dermaroller or the Dermapen® (Dermapen, Salt Lake City, UT, USA) [53, 54].

The standard medical dermaroller has a 12 cm–long handle with a 2 × 2 cm–wide drum-shaped cylinder at one end studded with 8 rows and 24 circular arrays of 192 fine microneedles, usually 0.5–3 mm in length and 0.1–0.25 mm in diameter [54]. These single-use microneedles are synthesized by reactive ion etching techniques on silicon or medical-grade stainless steel. The instrument is presterilized by gamma irradiation. Rolling with a standard dermaroller containing 192 needles of 2 mm length and 0.07 mm diameter 15 times over an area of skin results in approximately 250 holes per square centimeter up to the papillary dermis, depending on the pressure applied [55]. Each pass produces 16 micropunctures in the stratum corneum per square centimeter without damaging the epidermis significantly [53].

A simple dermaroller has evolved over the past decade through a variety of advancements. The current market is booming, with an assortment of devices based on needle length, drum size, and automation. The most important is the diversity of needle lengths. As noted in Chapter 1, a high ratio of tip length versus diameter of 13:1 is an important property of good needles [48]. For treating acne scars as a routine, a needle length of 1.5–2 mm is usually used. The minimum time interval between two sittings of microneedling depends the needle length of the dermaroller being used. The greater the needle length, greater should be the interval between sittings. When using 1.5 mm dermaroller, at least a three-week gap should be allowed between procedures [53].

Five basic types of medical dermarollers, which are registered with the FDA, have been described in the dermaroller series by Anastassakis, and most dermaroller devices are adapted from these elementary types [56].

- C-8 (cosmetic type), is the basic dermaroller as described earlier in this chapter, with a needle length of only 0.13 mm (130 µm) used for enhancing penetration of topical agents. It is completely painless.
- C-8HE (cosmetic type for hair-bearing surfaces, scalp) has a needle length of 0.2 mm (200 µm). Even this length is below the pain threshold.

- CIT-8 (medical type for collagen induction therapy) has a needle length of 0.5 mm (500 µm) and helps in collagen induction and skin remodeling.
- MF-8 (medical type) has a needle length of 1.5 mm (1500 µm). This creates deeper microchannels on the whole epidermis and dermis and at the same time destroys scar collagen bundles.
- MS-4 (medical type) is the only dermaroller that has a smaller cylinder, 1 cm length, 2 cm diameter, and subsequently four circular arrays of needles (for a total of 96 needles) 1.5 mm in length. It is used on areas where better precision and deeper penetration is required. It is mostly used on facial acne scars.

Home-care dermaroller

Home-care dermarollers (C-8) are used by patients themselves, as their needle length is below 0.15 mm. These are available for reduction of pore size and sebum production, as well as for transdermal delivery of products. Beauty Mouse® (Dermaroller Deutschland GmbH) is another approved device intended for home use [57]. It contains 480 needles of approximately 0.2 mm size, arranged on three separate drums, strategically placed inside a computer mouse–shaped device [57].

Other devices use additional technology to build upon the applications of mechanical MN. The Dermapen is an automated microneedling device which looks like a pen. This ergonomic device uses disposable needles and guides to adjust needle length for fractional mechanical resurfacing. The tip has 9–12 needles arranged in rows. It makes use of a rechargeable battery to operate in two modes – namely, the high-speed mode (700 cycles/min) and the low-speed mode (412 cycles/minute) in a vibrating stamplike manner [58]. It has the advantage of being reusable in different patients, as the needles are disposable; it's safe, as the needle tips are hidden inside the guide; and it includes the ability to easily adjust the needles' operating speeds and penetration depths, thereby permitting treatment of large surface areas efficiently and at varying needle depths as necessary for more convenient treatment of narrow areas such as the nose and around the eyes and lips without damaging the adjoining skin. This technology has been designed to overcome the issue of varying pressure as seen in manual dermarollers [41], thus making the procedure less painful [59].

Fractional radiofrequency microneedling

Recently a new technology has gained popularity. The amalgamation of microneedling with radiofrequency has further expanded the prospective applications of this technology. Insulated needles are used to penetrate the skin and release radiofrequency currents from the needle tips, producing thermal zones in the dermal structural

(a) (b)

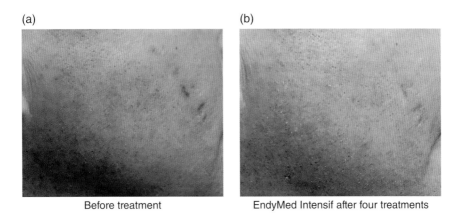

Before treatment   EndyMed Intensif after four treatments

Figure 6.1 A patient (a) before and (b) after treatment with MNRF. *Source:* Photos Courtesy of Michael H. Gold, MDGold Skin Care Center, The Laser and Rejuvenation Center, Nashville, TN.

components and accessory glands without damaging the overlying epidermis [60, 61]. This triggers long-term dermal remodeling, neoelastogenesis, and neocollagenesis. The depth of the needles can be adjusted from 0.5 mm to 3.5 mm, allowing clinicians to target different layers of the dermis discretely [61]. The operator can exercise good control over tissue damage by adjusting the power level and duration of the energy pulses.

The main energy-delivery system has a disposable tip with 49 gold-plated needles. Microneedling radiofrequency (MNRF) technology does not damage the epidermis, and is therefore safe in darker skin types [53]. There are many MNRF devices on the market, including Infini™ (Lutronic Co., Goyang-si, Korea), INTRAcel™ (Jeisys, Seoul, Korea), Vivace™ (Aesthetic Biomedical, USA) and Scarlet™ (ViOL, South Korea) fractional microneedling RF systems, and Intensif™ (ENDYMED, Israel). Figure 6.1 shows an example of a patient treated with fractional RF microneedling.

Light emitting microneedling device

LED microneedling rollers have been launched recently. These incorporate titanium microneedles [58]. These devices have not yet been explored and no published data is available regarding their efficacy.

Microneedle delivery systems

Microneedle delivery systems offer a minimally invasive and painless method of transdermal drug administration [62]. The various types of microneedles available for this purpose can be solid, coated, dissolving, hollow, and swellable polymer microneedles synthesized by microfabrication techniques [57]. Silicon, metals such as titanium, natural and synthetic polymers, and polysaccharides are the various materials used to fabricate these microneedles. Solid-coated microneedles are used to pierce the superficial skin, followed by topical application and delivery of the drug. Dissolvable or biodegradable and hollow needles deliver drugs directly into the dermis [62].

Discussion

Microneedling has been most extensively studied for acne scar treatment. Quite opposite to ablative lasers, the needles penetrate the epidermis but do not remove it; thus needling procedures can be safely performed without any downtime [29]. MN offers a relatively low=cost and minimally invasive treatment option. Apparently, the advantages of microneedling include not only a very low risk for postprocedural inflammatory hyperpigmentation but also a relatively short recovery period (two to three days), and a low cost [62].

A total of eight studies utilized microneedling in the treatment of postacne scarring. Treated scars were of various morphologic subtypes. In five papers, microneedling was used in isolation; in one it was compared with glycolic acid (GA) peeling; and in another it was used in conjunction with platelet-rich plasma (PRP) [63].

Fabbrocini et al. treated 32 patients with two sessions (eight weeks apart) of microneedling using a MS-4 dermaroller with 96 1.5 mm–long and 0.25 mm–wide needles [1]. Eight weeks after the first session, all patients had smoother facial skin and a slight reduction in scar severity. Eight weeks after the second session, there was evident improvement in scar appearance.

Microneedling has shown better results with combination treatments. One study compared the effects of microneedling to those of microneedling plus GA peeling [64]. Microneedling was performed every six weeks for five sessions with an MF-8 dermaroller (a drum-shaped device with 192 needles, each with a width of 0.25 mm and length of 1.5 mm) in group A, whereas group B underwent the same process of microneedling followed by a 35% GA peel three weeks later. The mean improvement in scars in group A was 31.33%, while that in group B was 62%.

Alam et al. performed a randomized, split-face, placebo-controlled clinical trial to investigate the effects of microneedling on various morphologic scar subtypes [65]. Fifteen individuals received three needling treatments that were performed at two-week intervals using an MTS roller, CR10 (1.0 mm) or CR20 (2.0 mm). Mean scar scores were significantly lower in the treatment group compared with baseline at six months. In the control group, mean scar scores did not vary significantly from baseline at three months and at six months. The mean pain rating was recorded as 1.08/10.

A further split-face study on 27 patients assessed the effects of microneedling with PRP versus microneedling with vitamin C application [66]. Microneedling was carried out with a 1.5 mm, 192-needle dermaroller. Scaring improvement was rated using the Goodman and Baron scale. An improvement by two grades was considered excellent, one grade was rated as good, and no change was labelled as a poor response. Twenty-three patients achieved reduction in scarring by one to two grades. Excellent response was seen in five (18.5%) patients with PRP, compared with two (7%) patients who received treatment with vitamin C.

One clinical trial by Dogra et al. evaluated the utility of microneedling for treating atrophic acne scars in Asian populations. They reviewed the response to five monthly sessions of dermaroller treatment in 30 patients with mixed types of atrophic acne scaring [28]. The equipment used was a 192-needle drum-shaped dermaroller with 1.5 mm–long and 0.1 mm–wide needles. The procedure was concluded when uniform pinpoint bleeding was achieved. At baseline, mean acne scar assessment scoring was 11.73 ± 3.12. At the five-month follow-up, the mean scoring had reduced to 6.5 ± 2.71. The mean scoring differences in patients with moderate and severe–grade scarring were 4.56 ± 1.31 and 6.00 ± 1.66, respectively. Four patients (13.3%) reported results as excellent, 20 (66.6%) as good, and six (20.0%) as poor.

Another study compared the effects of PRP to the CROSS peeling technique with 100% TCA versus combined microneedling and PRP in the treatment of atrophic acne scars. It showed significant improvement in the severity of acne scars after treatment ($P < 0.001$) in all three groups [67].

El-Domyati et al. evaluated the response of microneedling in 10 patients with different types of postacne atrophic scaring [29]. They used a dermaroller with 192 needles, 1.5 mm long and 0.25 mm wide. Patient satisfaction was documented to be 80–85% ($P = 0.001$). They quantified the histological changes induced by MN in 10 patients with atrophic facial scars from acne. Skin biopsies were obtained at baseline and post-treatment with the dermaroller [29]. There was a statistically significant increase in the production of collagen types I, III, and VII and a decrease in total elastin by the end of treatment ($p < 0.05$).

In a cohort study, Majid relied on clinical outcomes rather than histologic changes to assess improvement of atrophic facial scars in response to MN therapy [50]. Thirty-seven patients were offered dermaroller treatments and were followed for two months. Over 80% of the patients assessed their response to treatment as "excellent" on a 10-point scale, and 94.4% graded the reduction in the severity of their scars by at least one objective grade.

Several studies have also compared the efficacy of laser and MN treatments. Cachafeiro et al. compared 1,340 nm nonablative fractional erbium laser and Dr. Roller™ (Vydence Medical, São Carlos, São Paulo, Brazil) for the treatment of 46 patients with facial atrophic acne scars [68]. Both groups demonstrated improvement at two and six months post-treatment, with no statistically significant difference between them ($P = 0.264$). While efficacy was similar, patients who had undergone microneedling experienced erythema for an average of one day; patients who had undergone laser treatment experienced it for an average of three days. Additionally, 13.6% of the patients in the laser group experienced postinflammatory hyper/hypo-pigmentation (PIH) while none of the patients in the MN group did.

A clinical trial by Garg and Baveja assessed the efficacy of combination therapy using subcision, MN, and 15% trichloroacetic acid peel in the management of 50 patients with atrophic acne scars [69]. Patients were treated for a total of six sessions. Complete remission was demonstrated in all patients with Grade 2 scars and 22.7% of patients with Grade 3 scars. Additionally, out of the 16 patients with Grade 4 scars at baseline, 10 patients improved by two grades and the remaining 6 improved by one grade. Overall, 100% of patients had objective improvement in scars by at least one grade.

Pudukudan et al. reported the efficacy and safety of a noninsulated RF micronee-dling for in treating atrophic acne scars in patients with dark skin (Fitzpatrick skin types III to V) with minimal pain or downtime [70]. Chandrashekhar et al. conducted a study in 31 patients. Out of 13 patients with grade 4 scars, 12 patients (85.71%) showed improvement by 2 grades, i.e. their scars improved from grade 4 to grade 2 of Goodman and Baron scale. In 17 patients with grade 3 scars, 13 patients (76.47%) improved by 2 grades and 4 patients (23.52%) showed improvement by 1 grade [61].

Microneedling with fractional radiofrequency has also been studied for the treatment of active acne vulgaris. A study was performed on 18 patients with moderate to severe acne vulgaris with Fitzpatrick phototype IV to V skin. Two sessions of MFR were performed at a one-month interval. Sixteen patients showed objective clinical improvement, both in number and severity of inflammatory acne lesions. There was also an improvement in acne scars, enlarged facial pores, skin tone, and texture [71].

Another study was performed on 20 Korean patients with acne vulgaris. All of them received a single full-face MFR treatment. The casual sebum level and sebum excretion rate showed 30–60% and 70–80% reduction, respectively, two weeks post-treatment and remained below baseline until week eight, when the study ended [72].

In a prospective clinical trial, 25 patients with moderate to severe acne were treated with MFR. Results showed a decrease in the number of acne lesions (inflammatory and noninflammatory), though inflammatory lesions responded better than noninflammatory lesions [73].

Microneedle radio frequency systems deliver energy directly to the dermis via a number of microneedle electrodes and create a microthermal zone (MTZ), providing untouched areas between MTZs. With the advantages of the fractional energy delivery system of MFR devices and evidence of cytokine alteration, MNRF is helpful with offering less downtime in the treatment of acne vulgaris [73].

Conclusion

Microneedling therapy is a recent addition to the treatment armamentarium for managing acne and postacne scars. Since the development of the first dermaroller 20 years ago, a variety of new MN devices have been introduced. The treatment is performed as an in-office procedure after application of a local anesthetic cream, by means of a simple instrument such as a dermaroller, Dermapen, or other microneedling device. The needles cause small pinpoint injuries to the treated skin, which apparently heal within two to three days with no post-treatment sequelae. Microneedling treatment is becoming popular all over the world in the management of postacne scars because of the advantages this therapy offers over laser resurfacing; MN does not lead to any epidermal injury as is seen with lasers, giving an advantage of lesser risk of PIH in skin of color. There is minimal down-time associated with the procedure, unlike with ablative laser resurfacing, and the treatment is far more economical than laser treatments. Overall, MN offers a simple yet cost-effective therapeutic modality with minimal adverse events and a promising safety profile. Future large controlled clinical trials are imperative for the utility of this popular technique.

References

1 Fabbrocini G, Annunziata MC, D'Arco V, et al. Acne scars: pathogenesis, classification and treatment. Dermatol Res Pract. 2010:893080.
2 Williams C, Layton AM. Persistent acne in women: implications for the patient and for therapy. American Journal of Clinical Dermatology. 2006;7(5):281–290.
3 Strauss JS, Krowchuk DP, Leyden JJ, et al. Guidelines of care for acne vulgaris management. J Am Acad Dermatol. 2007;56(4):651–663. Epub 2007 Feb 5.
4 Abdel Hay R, Shalaby K, Zaher H, et al. Interventions for acne scars. Cochrane Database Syst. Rev. 2016;4(4):CD011946.
5 Collier CN, Harper JC, Cafardi JA, et al. The prevalence of acne in adults 20 years and older. J Am Acad Dermatol. 2008;58(1):56–59.
6 Jacob CI, Dover JS, Kaminer MS. Acne scarring: a classification system and review of treatment options. J Am Acad Dermatol. 2001;45:109–117.
7 Dalgard F, Gieler U, Holm JO, et al. Self-esteem and body satisfaction among late adolescents with acne: results from a population survey. Journal of the American Academy of Dermatology. 2009;59(5):746-751.
8 Conrado LA, Hounie AG, Diniz JB, et al. Body dysmorphic disorder among dermatologic patients: prevalence and clinical features. Journal of the American Academy of Dermatology. 2010;63(2):235–243.
9 Purvis D, Robinson E, Merry S, Watson P. Acne, anxiety, depression and suicide in teenagers: a cross-sectional survey of New Zealand secondary school students. J Paediatr Child Health. 2006;42(12):793–796.

10 Kurokawa I, Danby FW, Ju Q, et al. New developments in our understanding of acne pathogenesis and treatment. Experimental Dermatology. 2009;18(10):821–832.

11 Dreno B, Pecastaings S, Corvec S, et al. Cutibacterium acnes (Propionibacterium acnes) and acne vulgaris: a brief look at the latest updates. J Eur Acad Dermatol Venereol. 2018;32(Suppl 2):5–14.

12 Fitz-Gibbon S, Tomida S, Chiu BH, et al. Propionibacterium acnes strain populations in the human skin microbiome associated with acne. J Investig Dermatol. 2013;133: 2152–2160.

13 Kim J, Ochoa MT, Krutzik SR, et al. Activation of toll-like receptor 2 in acne triggers inflammatory cytokine responses. Journal of Immunology. 2002;169(3):1535–1541.

14 Wolfram D, Tzankov A, P¨ulzl P, Piza-Katzer H. Hypertrophic scars and keloids—a review of their pathophysiology, risk factors, and therapeutic management. Dermatol Surgery. 2009;35(2):171–181.

15 Cowin AJ, Brosnan MP, Holmes TM, Ferguson MWJ. Endogenous inflammatory response to dermal wound healing in the fetal and adult mouse. Dev Dyn. 1998;212(3):385–393.

16 Stadelmann WK, Digenis AG, Tobin GR. Physiology and healing dynamics of chronic cutaneous wounds. American Journal of Surgery. 1998;176(2A):26S–38S.

17 Baum CL, Arpey CJ. Normal cutaneous wound healing: clinical correlation with cellular and molecular events. Dermatol Surg. 2005;31(6):674–686.

18 Midwood KS, Williams LV, Schwarzbauer JE. Tissue repair and the dynamics of the extracellular matrix. Int J Biochem Cell Biol. 2004;36(6):1031–1037.

19 Holland DB, Jeremy AHT, Roberts SG, et al. Inflammation in acne scarring: a comparison of the responses in lesions from patients prone and not prone to scar. Br J Dermatol. 2004;150(1):72–81.

20 Martin P, Leibovich SJ. Inflammatory cells during wound repair: the good, the bad and the ugly. Trends in Cell Biology. 2005;5(11):599–607.

21 Patel MJ, Antony A, Do T, et al. Atrophic acne scars may arise from both inflammatory and non-inflammatory acne lesions. 2010 Annual Meeting of the Society for Investigative Dermatology, Atlanta, GA United States.

22 Jordan RE, Cummins CL, Burls AJ, Seukeran DC. Laser resurfacing for facial acne scars. Cochrane Database Syst. Rev. 2001;1.

23 Layton AM, Henderson CA, Cunliffe WJ. A clinical evaluation of acne scarring and its incidence. Clin Exp Dermatol. 1994;19(4):303–308. [MEDLINE: 7955470].

24 Goodman GJ, Baron JA. Postacne scarring—a quantitative global scarring grading system. J Cosmet Dermatol. 2006;5(1):48–52.

25 Basta-Juzbasic A. Current therapeutic approach to acne scars. Acta Dermatovenerologica Croatica. 2010;18(3):171–175.

26 Maibach HI, Gorouhi F. Evidence Based Dermatology. People's Medical Publishing House; Shelton, CT: 2011.

27 Chivot M, Pawin H, Beylot C, et al. Acne scars: epidemiology, physiopathology, clinical features and treatment. Annales de Dermatologie et de Venereologie. 2006;133(10): 813–824.

28 Dogra S, Yadav S, Sarangal R. Microneedling for acne scars in Asian skin type: an effective low cost treatment modality. J Cosmet Dermatol. 2014;13(3):180–187.

29 El-Domyati M, Barakat M, Awad S, et al. Microneedling therapy for atrophic acne scars: an objective evaluation. J Clin Aesthet Dermatol. 2015;8:36–42.

30 Lee JB, Chung WG, Kwahck H, Lee KH. Focal treatment of acne scars with trichloro-acetic acid: chemical reconstruction of skin scars method. Dermatol Surg. 2002;28:1017–1021.

31 Levy LL, Zeichner JA. Management of acne scarring, part II: a comparative review of non-laser-based, minimally invasive approaches. Am J Clin Dermatol. 2012;13: 331–340.

32 Weber MB, Machado RB, Hoefel IR, et al. Complication of CROSS-technique on boxcar acne scars: atrophy. Dermatol Surg. 2011;37:93–95.

33 Gold MH. Dermabrasion in dermatology. Am J Clin Dermatol. 2003;4:467–471.

34 Bolognia J, Jorizzo JL, Schaffer JV. Dermatology (3rd ed). Elsevier Saunders; Philadelphia, PA: 2012.

35 Karnik J, Baumann L, Bruce S, et al. A double-blind, randomized, multicenter, con-trolled trial of suspended polymethylmethacrylate microspheres for the correction of atrophic facial acne scars. J Am Acad Dermatol. 2014;71(1):77–83.

36 Hasson A, Romero WA. Treatment of facial atrophic scars with Esthelis, a hyaluronic acid filler with polydense cohesive matrix (CPM). J Drugs Dermatol. 2010;9: 1507–1509.

37 Hedelund L, Moreau KE, Beyer DM, et al. Fractional nonablative 1,540-nm laser resur-facing of atrophic acne scars. A randomized controlled trial with blinded response evaluation. Lasers Med Sci. 2010;25(5):749–754.

38 Goel A, Krupashankar DS, Aurangabadkar S, et al. Fractional lasers in dermatology—current status and recommendations. Indian J Dermatol Venereol Leprol. 2011;77(3): 369–379.

39 Alexiades-Armenakas MR, Dover JS, Arndt KA. Fractional laser skin resurfacing. J Drugs Dermatol. 2012;11(11):1274–1287.

40 Rinaldi F. Laser: a review. Clin Dermatol. 2008;26(6):590–601.

41 Alster TS, Graham PM. Microneedling: a review and practical guide. Dermatol Surg. 2018;44(3):397–404.

42 Doddaballapur S. Microneedling with dermaroller. J Cutan Aesthet Surg. 2009;2: 110–111.

43 Habbema L, Verhagen R, Van Hal R, et al. Minimally invasive non-thermal laser tech-nology using laser-induced optical breakdown for skin rejuvenation. J Biophotonics. 2012;5:194–199.

44 Orentreich DS, Orentreich N. Subcutaneous incisionless (subcision) surgery for the correction of depressed scars and wrinkles. Dermatol Surg. 1995;21:543–549.

45 Camirand A, Doucet J. Needle dermabrasion. Aesth Plast Surg. 1997;21:48–51.

46 Fernandes D. Percutaneous collagen induction: an alternative to laser resurfacing. Aesthet Surg J. 2002;22:307–309.

47 Aust MC, Fernandes D, Kolokythas P, et al. Percutaneous collagen induction therapy: an alternative treatment for scars, wrinkles and skin laxity. Plast Reconstr Surg. 2008;121:1421–1429.

48 Nair PA, Arora TH. Microneedling using dermaroller: a means of collagen induction therapy. GMJ. 2014;69:24–27.

49 Liebl H, Kloth LC. Skin cell proliferation stimulated by microneedles. J Am Coll Clin Wound Spec. 2012;4:2.

50 Majid I, Sheikh G, September PI. Microneedling and its applications in dermatology. In Prime. 2014;4(7):44–49.

51 Jaffe L. Control of development by steady ionic currents. Fed Proc. 1981;40:125–127.

52 Kloth LC. Electrical stimulation for wound healing: A review of evidence from in vitro studies, animal experiments, and clinical trials. Int J Low Extrem Wounds. 2005;4:23–44.

53 Singh A, Yadav S. Microneedling: advances and widening horizons. Indian Dermatol Online J. 2016;7(4):244–254.

54 Bahuguna A. Microneedling-facts and fictions. Asian J Med Sci. 2013;4:1–4.

55 Bhardwaj D. Collagen induction therapy with dermaroller. Community Based Med J. 2013;1:35–37.

56 Anastassakis K. The Dermaroller Series. http://www.mtoimportadora.com.br/site_novo/wp-content/uploads/2014/04/Dr.-Anastassakis-Kostas.pdf.

57 McCrudden MT, McAlister E, Courtenay AJ, et al. Microneedle applications in improving skin appearance. Exp Dermatol. 2015;24(8):561–566.

58 Arora S, Gupta BP. Automated microneedling device–a new tool in dermatologist's kit–a review. J Pak Med Assoc. 2012;22:354–357.

59 Lewis W. Is microneedling really the next big thing? Wendy Lewis explores the buzz surrounding skin needling. Plast Surg Pract. 2014;7:24–28.

60 Cohen BE, Elbuluk N. Microneedling in skin of color: a review of uses and efficacy. J Am Acad Dermatol. 2016;74:348–355.

61 Chandrashekar BS, Sriram R, Mysore R, et al. Evaluation of microneedling fractional radiofrequency device for treatment of acne scars. J Cutan Aesthet Surg. 2014;7:93–97.

62 Bariya SH, Gohel MC, Mehta TA, Sharma OP. Microneedles: an emerging transdermal drug delivery system. J Pharm Pharmacol. 2012;64:11–29.

63 Kravvas G, Al-Niaimi F. A systematic review of treatments for acne scarring. Part 1: Non-energy-based techniques. Scars Burn Heal. 2017;3.

64 Sharad J. Combination of microneedling and glycolic acid peels for the treatment of acne scars in dark skin. J Cosmet Dermatol. 2011;10:317–323.

65 Alam M, Han S, Pongprutthipan M, et al. Efficacy of a needling device for the treatment of acne scars: a randomized clinical trial. JAMA Dermatol. 2014;150:844–849.

66 Chawla S. Split face comparative study of microneedling with PRP versus microneedling with vitamin C in treating atrophic post acne scars. J Cutan Aesthet Surg. 2014;7:209–212.

67 Nofal E, Helmy A, Nofal A, et al. Platelet-rich plasma versus CROSS technique with 100% trichloroacetic acid versus combined skin needling and platelet rich plasma in the treatment of atrophic acne scars: a comparative study. Dermatol Surg. 2014;40:864–873.

68 Cachafeiro T, Escobar G, Maldonado G, et al. Comparison of nonablative fractional erbium laser 1,340 nm and microneedling for the treatment of atrophic acne scars: a randomized clinical trial. Dermatol Surg. 2016;42(2):232–241.

69 Garg S, Baveja S. Combination therapy in the management of atrophic acne scars. J Cutan Aesthet Surg. 2014;7(1):18–23.

70 David Pudukadan. Treatment of acne scars on darker skin types using a non insulated smooth motion, electronically controlled radiofrequency microneedles treatment system. Dermatol Surg. 2017;43:S64–S69.

71 Lee SB. The treatment of burn scar-induced contracture with the pinhole method and collagen induction therapy: a case report. J Eur Acad Dermatol Venereol. 2008;22: 513–514.

72 Lee KR, Lee EG, Lee HJ, Yoon MS. Assessment of treatment efficacy and sebosuppressive effect of fractional radiofrequency microneedle on acne vulgaris. Lasers Surg Med. 2013;45:639–647.

73 Kim ST, Lee KH, Sim HJ, et al. Treatment of acne vulgaris with fractional radiofrequency microneedling. J Dermatol. 2014;41:586–591.

7 Microneedling and Platelet-Rich Plasma (PRP)

Elizabeth Bahar Houshmand

Houshmand Dermatology and Wellness, Dallas, TX, USA

Introduction

As discussed in earlier chapters of this textbook, microneedling (also known as collagen induction therapy or percutaneous collagen induction) is an increasingly popular treatment modality for skin rejuvenation. The approach employs small needles to puncture the skin and stimulate local collagen production in a minimally invasive manner (see Figure 7.1).

It has been utilized in aesthetic medicine for many years and is an excellent therapeutic option for multiple indications.

In recent years, microneedling has been combined with platelet-rich plasma (PRP) with the aim of augmenting cosmetic outcomes. It has been used alone and for optimization in a number of clinical indications, including but not limited to skin rejuvenation, alopecia treatment, and notably acne scarring.

This chapter will discuss PRP and its use in combination therapies with microneedling.

Platelet-rich plasma – what is it?

PRP is an autologous high concentration of platelets derived from blood plasma. It contains numerous growth factors, such as PGF, TGFβ, EGF, VEGF, FGF, and insulinlike GF (see Table 7.1), and multiple cytokines that stimulate collagen and wound healing [1]. The combination of PRP with other dermatologic procedures

Microneedling: Global Perspectives in Aesthetic Medicine, First Edition.
Edited by Elizabeth Bahar Houshmand.
© 2021 John Wiley & Sons Ltd. Published 2021 by John Wiley & Sons Ltd.

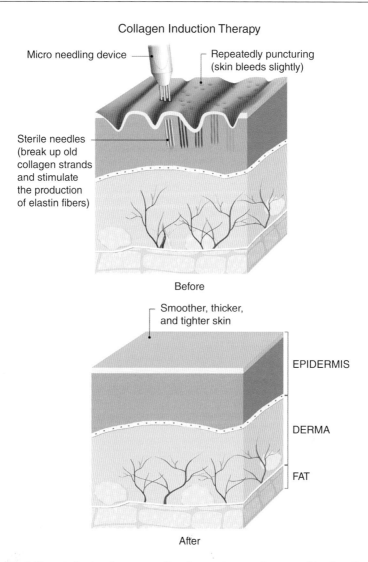

Figure 7.1 Collagen induction therapy: needling forms minute perforations of the skin. This results in both superficial capillary and dermal microinjuries, leading to growth factor release and fibroblast infiltration. *Source:* designua/123RF.

intended for skin and hair health and treatments may offer benefits in the form of reduced downtime and better efficacy. PRP applied to the skin post-microneedling with roller, stamp, or pen has a mechanically induced altered epidermal barrier. PRP has been applied topically or injected into the skin after microneedling to enhance the outcomes and decrease the downtime from these procedures.

Table 7.1 All the growth factors.

Name	Abbreviation	Function
Platelet-derived growth factor	PDGF	Enhances collagen synthesis, proliferation of bone cells, fibroblast chemotaxis and proliferative activity, and macrophage activation
Transforming growth factor-β	TGF-β	Enhances synthesis of type I collagen, promotes angiogenesis, stimulates chemotaxis of immune cells, and inhibits osteoclast formation and bone resorption
Vascular endothelial growth factor	VEGF	Stimulates angiogenesis, migration and mitosis of endothelial cells, increases permeability of the vessels, and stimulates chemotaxis of macrophages and neutrophils
Epidermal growth factor	EGF	Stimulates cellular proliferation and differentiation of epithelial cells; promotes cytokine secretion by mesenchymal and epithelial cells
Insulinlike growth factor	IGF	Promotes cell growth, differentiation, and recruitment in bone, blood vessel, skin and other tissues; stimulates collagen synthesis together with PDGF
Fibroblast growth factor	FGF	Promotes proliferation of mesenchymal cells, chondrocytes and osteoblasts; stimulates the growth and differentiation of chondrocytes and osteoblasts

Source: Pavlovic, V., Ciric, M., Jovanovic, V., & Stojanovic, P. (2016). Platelet Rich Plasma: a short overview of certain bioactive components. *Open Medicine, 11*(1). © 2016, De Gruyter.

Combination therapy

Microneedling provides accelerated neocollagenesis. Collagen induction therapy, in combination with the additional growth factors and cytokines from PRP, may act synergistically with the microneedling cascade to provide enhanced collagen remodeling and patient outcomes.

History of PRP

PRP has been utilized for many years in dentistry, orthopedics, endodentistry, and other surgical fields. In recent years, it has been added to the fields of plastic surgery and dermatology and has been used for aesthetic medicine treatments. Literature reviews have been conducted regarding the use of PRP for cosmetic rejuvenation and augmentation. In 2017, Frautschi et al. published a comprehensive review searching for reports of PRP in aesthetic medicine published from 1950 to 2015 [2]. The authors reviewed 38 reports and concluded that the published studies produced promising results but there was a lack of standardized protocols in preparation, composition, and activation methods of the PRP, making reproducible scientific outcomes difficult. A review of PRP in aesthetic medicine from 2006 to 2015 by Motosko et al agreed; although the studies had positive outcomes, significant protocol variation existed in preparation and treatment protocols for PRP, which makes reproducible and standardized treatment recommendations a challenge [3].

Because PRP is autologous, there is innate variability in the PRP platelet concentration. Platelet concentrations in adults has a normal variable range from 150,000 to 450,000/ uL, and this can impact the PRP concentration by threefold. To date, there are no standardized protocols established by a large-scale study analyzing baseline values of patients platelet counts and treatment outcomes based on these findings.

The initial findings are promising, but more evidence-based standardized research methods and protocols are needed to provide guidance for PRP protocols in aesthetic practices (see Figure 7.2).

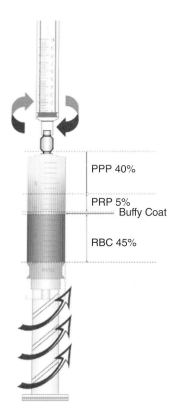

Figure 7.2 Makeup of PRP: PPP, PRP, and RBC. Plasma: 55–91% water, 7% proteins, 2% electrolytes. Buffy coat: 1% -Wbc, platelets. RBC: 99% of total volume.

The PRP microneedling procedure

Microneedling combination therapy with PRP is an in-office procedure. It begins with thorough cleansing and preparation of the skin and topical anesthetic application to the treatment areas. Then the patient's blood is drawn and centrifuged, and the PRP is extracted. After removal of the numbing cream and thorough cleansing of the skin, microneedling begins and the PRP is applied immediately to deeply penetrate the new micro-opening channels in the skin. I recommend immediate application, as the microchannels are only open for a very brief duration of time. Additionally, direct pore injections of PRP can be utilized to target hyperpigmentation and for textural improvement especially for pore size and superficial rhytides.

The micro-openings are thought to close rapidly, approximately 10–15 minutes after needling is performed [4]. Minor side effects may include erythema lasting approximately three to five days. Some patients also experience mild edema after the procedure, which tends to subside along with the erythema. Most side effects are non-lasting. The procedure is done with minimal discomfort or pain. Results are not immediate; they typically are visible within three to four weeks after the procedure (Figure 7.3). For most patients, depending on the indicated treatment

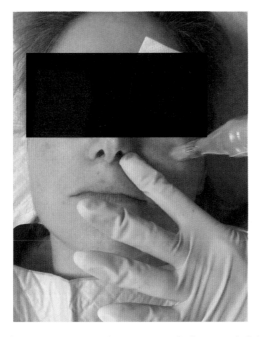

Figure 7.3 PRP for skin rejuvenation. Gentle traction is applied, in a sterile field, while the microneedle tip is held perpendicular to the skin's surface in order to allow a smooth surface for the microneedles to penetrate the skin evenly. *Source:* Elizabeth Bahar Houshmand MD.

plan, the patient's condition, and outcomes desired, three or four sessions scheduled at approximately four-week intervals is the current recommendation.

Indications

Acne scars

Acne scarring causes cosmetic discomfort, depression, low self-esteem, and reduced quality of life. Microneedling is an established treatment for acne scars, most notably atrophic scars (Figure 7.4), although the efficacy of PRP has not been thoroughly explored. There are several studies looking at the combination therapy both in terms of therapeutic outcomes and cost benefit for the treatments.

Atrophic scarring is a consequence of abnormal resolution or wound healing following acne inflammation. They are broadly classified as macular, atrophic, and hypertrophic or keloidal scars. Atrophic acne scars are further divided into three types: icepick, boxcar, and rolling scars [5].

Three studies, discussed in this section, looked at acne scar treatments in relation to therapy with and without the combination therapy of microneedling and PRP.

Asif et al. compared two groups of patients with acne scars. In total, 50 patients were treated: group one received microneedling treatments with PRP (PRP MN) and group two received microneedling and distilled water sessions. Both groups showed some improvement in scars; however, the PRP MN group showed a 62.2% improvement while the microneedling with distilled water subjects had only a 45.84% improvement. These results support the increased benefits of PRP MN combination therapy vs. microneedling alone [6].

(a)   (b)

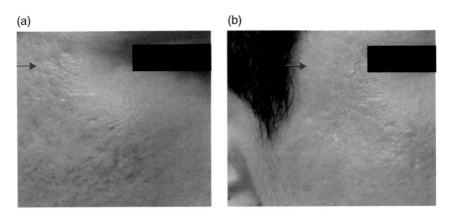

Figure 7.4 Acne scarring at (a) baseline and (b) three months after three needling sessions. *Source:* Elizabeth Bahar Houshmand MD.

Chawla compared the effectiveness of combination therapy with microneedling plus PRP versus microneedling and vitamin C application [7]. A total of 27 patients completed the treatment schedules over a six-month period, with an interval of one month between the vitamin C and PRP treatments. Each patient received four treatments of PRP MN on one side of the face and MN with vitamin C on the other side. Patients who participated in the PRP study reported a higher incidence of favorable results when compared to the group that tested with vitamin C. Twenty-one patients (78%) patients experienced good to excellent results from the PRP MN vs. 17 (63%) of the MN with vitamin C patients. PRP with microneedling had superior results in comparison to microneedling with vitamin C.

Of note, assessments of improvement were performed by the treating physician and patient satisfaction reports were completed with knowledge of the therapies and cost factors, which may have influenced results [7].

In another split-face study, Fabbrocini et al. evaluated 12 adult patients with acne scars [8]. The right side of their faces received microneedling plus PRP, while the left side received microneedling alone. Two treatments were performed eight weeks apart. Severity scores (0 = no lesions; 10 = maximum severity) were used to assess patient outcomes throughout the study. Acne scars improved on both sides of the face following the treatment period, but the reduction in scar severity with microneedling plus PRP (3.5 points) was significantly greater than with microneedling alone (2.6 points) – $P<.05$. Patients tended to experience two or three days of mild swelling and erythema after treatment, regardless of PRP addition. With only

(a)   (b)

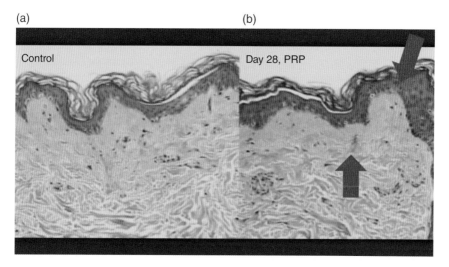

Figure 7.5 (a) Histologic image showing a thin epidermis and flattened rete ridges and collagen in parallel bundles. (b) Histologic image showing the results at day 28 after treatment with PRP. Note the thickened epidermis and normal rete ridges with the beautiful wavy pink thickened collagen bundles in a lattice pattern.

12 patients, the study was limited by a small sample size. The 10-point grading system differed from the Goodman and Baron scale in that it lacked corresponding qualitative markers, likely decreasing reproducibility [9].

Treatment with microneedling in acne patients and for other indications promotes skin rejuvenation by creating small puncture wounds in the epidermis and dermis. This injury triggers the wound-healing cascade and alters the modulation of growth factors to promote regenerative effects [10, 11]. Following microneedling therapy, increases occur in elastic fiber formation, collagen deposition, and dermal thickness [12]. Of interesting histologic note, collagen is deposited in the normal lattice pattern following this treatment rather than in the parallel bundles typical of scars (see Figure 7.5) [13].

Alopecia

Hair plays an important role in identity, self-perception, and psychosocial functioning. Hair loss can be a devastating experience that decreases self-esteem and feelings of personal attractiveness while also leading to depression and anxiety [14, 15]. Patients are seeking effective procedures with reduced downtimes.

Platelet-rich plasma – monotherapy and alopecia treatment

PRP as monotherapy has demonstrated significant improvements in hair growth when treating androgenic alopecia (AGA) in dermatology (See Table 7.2). PRP growth factors promote hair regrowth by stimulating stem cell differentiation of hair follicles, inducing and prolonging the proliferative anagen phase of hair follicles, as well as activating antiapoptotic pathways and promoting angiogenesis to increase perifollicular vascularization and the survival of dermal papilla fibroblasts (Table 7.2) [15, 16–18]. Platelet-rich plasma is derived from the supernatant of centrifuged whole blood and then injected into the dermis of the scalp to stimulate hair growth.

Although use of PRP is not approved or cleared by the FDA for treatment of hair loss, several studies have demonstrated the efficacy of autologous PRP use for treating AGA [19]. One pilot study of 19 male and female participants given a total of five PRP injections monthly for three months and subsequently at months four and seven found a statistically significant improvement in mean hair density, hair diameter, and terminal-vellus hair ratio at the one-year follow-up. Furthermore, histomorphometric evaluation demonstrated a decrease in perivascular inflammatory infiltrate [20].

Several studies indicate that PRP is a promising treatment for thinning hair [2]. Both male and female pattern hair loss, as well as alopecia areata, can be improved with PRP. A trial of 40 men and women found that subdermal PRP injections

Table 7.2 Importance of alpha granules in hair loss.

Granule Type	Mediator Examples	Role
Adhesion modules	Fibrinogen	Leukocyte adhesion
Chemokines	CXCL-1, 4, 5, 7, 8CCL-2, 3, 5	WBC recruitment
Cytokines	IL-1β	Antigen presentation
Growth factors	PDGF, TGG-β	Would healing, immune modulation
Microbial proteins	Kinocidins, Defensins, Throm bocidins	Antimicrobial peptides

administered three times per month, with booster injections administered three months later, was more effective than other injection regimens, including once-monthly injections [21, 22]. Activators such as collagen, thrombin, 10% calcium chloride, and calcium gluconate may be added to the PRP serum to promote further growth factor secretion upon platelet activation [23]. However, different means of activation are used in different trials, potentially leading to varying results in clinical trials, with no one proven superior method [24–26].

Studies using an insufficient number of treatments lacked substantial improvements [27]. Multiple continued treatments with PRP are necessary for significant aesthetic improvement of increased hair density. It is thought that three injections spaced 8–12 weeks apart each year is the minimum frequency in order to observe any clinically beneficial result (see Figure 7.6).

In clinical practice, most physicians commence with a series of monthly injections for three to four sessions, then continue with maintenance therapies once every six months (twice a year). This will vary based on the patient's response and physicians have used monthly treatments for up to six sessions with a more frequent maintenance regimen. This is dependent on the patient's clinical response, which is influenced by multiple factors: age, genetics, stress level, and overall health. More research is needed to determine proper frequency, dosing, and maintenance protocols to optimize results.

The main drawback of PRP use is that there is no consensus regarding exact concentration, utility of activators, dosing parameters, depth of injection, or frequency of sessions [23]. Transient pain and erythema are the most common side effects of PRP injections, with no major adverse effects reported in the literature [27].

Microneedling

Microneedling also has shown promise in treating androgenic alopecia, increasing hair regrowth in patients who previously showed poor response to conventional therapy with minoxidil and finasteride [11, 12]. PRP is developed by enriching

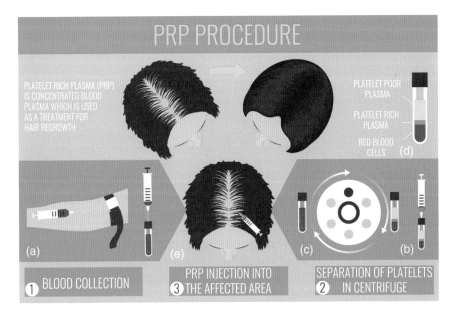

Figure 7.6 Steps for PRP collection in a single-spin method. (a) Blood collection venipuncture from antecubital vein. (b) Transfer of blood into collection tube for centrifugation. (c) Placement of specimen in centrifuge. (d) Withdrawal of the test tube that has the PPP, PRP, and RBC to withdraw the PRP for injection. (e) Subdermal injection of PRP into the scalp. *Source:* art4stock/ Shutterstock.com.

blood with an autologous concentration of platelets. The typical platelet count of whole blood is approximately 200,000/µL; PRP aims to prepare a platelet count of at least 1,000,000/µL in a 5 mL volume [14]. The key component of PRP is its high concentration of growth factors, including platelet-derived growth factor, transforming growth factor, vascular endothelial growth factor, and epithelial growth factor [15].

Microneedling is proposed to increase hair regrowth by triggering the wound-healing response, which ultimately augments the release of platelet-derived and epidermal growth factors while also activating the hair bulge [28]. Treatment often is performed with a roller instrument that uses needles 0.5–2.5 mm long. Topical anesthetic cream may be applied prior to treatment [29]. The treated area is then washed and an antibiotic ointment is applied [30]. Management regimens typically require daily to weekly treatments, with a total of 12 to 28 weeks to demonstrate an effect.

Microneedling has demonstrated efficacy in the treatment of hair loss, especially when combined with minoxidil. One study randomized 68 patients to undergo microneedling with minoxidil solution 5% twice daily, compared to a control group of minoxidil solution 5% twice daily alone. After 12 weeks, patients treated with microneedling and minoxidil had significantly higher hair counts than the control group ($P<.05$) [31]. It is speculated that microneedling increases penetration of topical medications, including minoxidil, across the skin barrier, thereby enhancing absorption of large molecules [28].

Combination of microneedling and PRP

Topical PRP has been used synergistically to augment the effects of microneedling. A trial randomized 93 patients with alopecia to receive minoxidil solution 5% alone, minoxidil solution 5% plus PRP, or microneedling with PRP. Hair growth was appreciated in 26 of 31 patients treated with microneedling and PRP [32, 33], compared to 10 of 31 and 17 of 31 in the other two groups, respectively. However, when hair growth occurred in the minoxidil-treated group, it occurred faster, with changes in hair growth at 12 weeks compared to 26 weeks in the microneedling group. When evaluating the efficacy of microneedling and PRP, it must be noted that there is no established leading protocol for treating hair loss, which may affect the success of the treatment.

Combination therapy: alopecia areata treatment

Hair loss affects millions of Americans each year and has detrimental effects on self-esteem and psychosocial functioning. Treatment options are emerging, including the use of PRP and microneedling.

Platelet-rich plasma and microneedling have been investigated recently as potential therapeutic options for the treatment of hair loss and hair disorders. Evidence from laboratory studies indicates that these treatments enhance growth factor production that, in turn, facilitates hair follicle development and cycling which is useful for the treatment of alopecia areata.

A subset of patients with alopecia areata respond insufficiently to the conventionally available treatments and consequently seek alternative therapeutic options [34]. Microneedling is also hypothesized to enhance growth factors while augmenting collagen and elastin production and creating microchannels that allow for transdermal delivery of drugs through the stratum corneum [35].

This technique has similarly been evaluated for the treatment of androgenetic alopecia with promising results, and may have applications for the treatment of other hair disorders [30].

Although the exact mechanism of PRP has not been fully resolved, strong evidence suggests that PRP increases concentrations of growth factors, cytokines, and proteins, thereby modulating inflammatory pathways and tissue repair [36]. During the wound-healing process, platelets become activated and release the contents of alpha granules that contain platelet-derived growth factor, transforming growth factor-ß, vascular endothelial growth factor, epidermal growth factor, and insulinlike growth factor-1 [37]. See the following list of growth factors in platelet alpha granules.

- Platelet-derived growth factor α and β (PDGF-α and -β)
- Transforming growth factor-β (TGFβ) 1 & 2
- Platelet factor 4
- Vascular endothelial growth factor (VEGF)
- Insulinlike growth factor-1 (IGF-1)
- Interleukin-1 (IL-1)
- Hepatocyte growth factor
- Platelet-derived endothelial growth factor
- Epithelial cell growth factor
- Fibroblast growth factor (FGF)

A study conducted by Eppley et al. in 2004 examined the composition of PRP taken from 10 patients ranging in age from 29 to 58 years [38]. In terms of growth factors, platelet-derived growth factor, transforming growth factor-ß, vascular endothelial growth factor, and epidermal growth factor were all significantly increased in the platelet-rich blood relative to whole blood baseline samples.

Another study using Ki-67 as a marker of cellular proliferation similarly identified significantly higher levels in hair removed from patients treated with PRP [39]. Together these results suggest that PRP may enhance proliferation of cells in the hair follicle and help patients with alopecia areata recalcitrant to other therapies.

Conclusion

PRP and microneedling continue to evolve as therapeutic tools in dermatology and aesthetic medicine. Numerous growth factors contained within PRP promote neocollagenesis, angiogenesis, and overall proliferation of stem cells and soft tissue remodeling. PRP is easily harvested from patients' own whole blood using numerous commercially available systems, making it a safe in-office procedure. Top evidence-based dermatologic indications for microneedling and PRP include hair restoration and skin rejuvenation, as well as improvements in acne scars. Combination therapy of PRP with microneedling has demonstrated synergistic effects, enhancing overall cosmetic outcomes. The dermatologic community stresses that more studies are needed to further standardize and define PRP protocols for specific indications. Nonsurgical treatments continue to offer patients multiple options, as they are often less costly and do not carry the same risks and downtime associated with surgical procedures. This is an exciting area of growth in the field of cosmetic medicine, offering improved results for our patients.

References

1 Lubkowska A, Dolegowska B, Banfi G. Growth factor content in PRP and their applicability in medicine. J Biol Regul Homeost Agents. 2012;26(2 suppl 1):3S-22S.

2 Russell S. Frautschi BS, Hashem AM, et al. Current Evidence for Clinical Efficacy of Platelet Rich Plasma in Aesthetic Surgery: A Systematic Review. Aesthet Surg J. 2017;37(3):353–362.

3 Motosko CC, Khouri KS, Poudrier G, et al. Evaluating platelet-rich therapy for facial aesthetics and alopecia: a critical review of the literature. Plast Reconstr Surg. 2018;141:1115–1123.

4 Fernandes D, Signorini M. Combating photoaging with percutaneous collagen induction. Clin Dermatol. 2008;26:192–199.

5 Camirand A, Doucet J. Needle dermabrasion. Aesthetic Plast Surg. 1997;21:48–51.

6 Asif M, Kanodia S, Singh K. Combined autologous platelet-rich plasma with microneedling verses microneedling with distilled water in the treatment of atrophic acne scars: a concurrent split-face study. J Cosmet Dermatol. 2016;15:434–443.

7 Chawla S. Split face comparative study of microneedling with PRP versus microneedling with vitamin C in treating atrophic post acne scars. J Cutan Aesthet Surg. 2014;7:209–212.

8 Fabbrocini G, De Vita V, Pastore F, et al. Combined use of skin needling and platelet-rich plasma in acne scarring treatment. J Cosmet Dermatol. 2011;24:177–183.

9 Goodman GJ, Baron JA. Postacne scarring: a qualitative global scarring grading system. Dermatol Surg. 2006;32:1458–1466.

10 Fabbrocini G, Fardella N, Monfrecola A, et al. Acne scarring treatment using skin needling. Clin Exp Dermatol. 2009;34:874–879.

11 Zeitter S, Sikora Z, Jahn S, et al. Microneedling: matching the results of medical needling and repetitive treatments to maximize potential for skin regeneration. Burns. 2014;40:966–973.

12 Schwarz M, Laaff H. A prospective controlled assessment of microneedling with the Dermaroller device. Plast Reconstr Surg. 2011;127:E146-E148.

13 Fernandes D, Signorini M. Combating photoaging with percutaneous collagen induction. Clin Dermatol. 2008;26:192–199.

14 Saed S, Ibrahim O, Bergfeld WF. Hair camouflage: a comprehensive review. Int J Womens Dermatol. 2016;2:122–127.

15 Alfonso M, Richter-Appelt H, Tosti A, et al. The psychosocial impact of hair loss among men: a multinational European study. Curr Med Res Opin. 2005;21:1829–1836.

16 Messenger AG, Rundegren J. Minoxidil: mechanisms of action on hair growth. Br J Dermatol. 2004;150:186–194.

17 Mori O, Uno H. The effect of topical minoxidil on hair follicular cycles of rats. J Dermatol. 1990;17:276–281.

18 Pekmezci E, Turkoglu M, Gokalp H, et al. Minoxidil downregulates interleukin-1 alpha gene expression in HaCaT cells. Int J Trichol. 2018;10:108–112.

19 Jha AK, Vinay K, Zeeshan M, et al. Platelet-rich plasma and microneedling improves hair growth in patients of androgenetic alopecia when used as an adjuvant to minoxidil. J Cosmet Dermatol. doi:10.1111/jocd.12864.

20 Anitua E, Pino A, Martinez N, et al. The effect of plasma rich in growth factors on pattern hair loss: a pilot study. Dermatol Surg. 2017;43:658–670.

21 Puig CJ, Reese R, Peters M. Double-blind, placebo-controlled pilot study on the use of platelet-rich plasma in women with female androgenetic alopecia. Dermatol Surg. 2016;42:1243–1247.

22 Mapar MA, Shahriari S, Haghighizadeh MH. Efficacy of platelet-rich plasma in the treatment of androgenetic (male-patterned) alopecia: a pilot randomized controlled trial. J Cosmet Laser Ther. 2016;18:452–455.

23 Maria-Angeliki G, Alexandros-Efstratios K, Dimitris R, et al. Platelet-rich plasma as a potential treatment for noncicatricial alopecias. Int J Trichol. 2015;7:54–63.

24 Gkini MA, Kouskoukis AE, Tripsianis G, et al. Study of platelet-rich plasma injections in the treatment of androgenetic alopecia through an one-year period. J Cutan Aesthet Surg. 2014;7:213–219.

25 Landesberg R, Roy M, Glickman RS. Quantification of growth factor levels using a simplified method of platelet-rich plasma gel preparation. J Oral Maxillofac Surg. 2000;58:297–300; discussion 300–301.

26 Weibrich G, Kleis WK, Hafner G. Growth factor levels in the platelet-rich plasma produced by 2 different methods: curasan-type PRP kit versus PCCS PRP system. Int J Oral Maxillofac Implants. 2002;17:184–190.

27 Alves R, Grimalt R. Randomized placebo-controlled, double-blind, half-head study to assess the efficacy of platelet-rich plasma on the treatment of androgenetic alopecia. Dermatol Surg. 2016;42:491–497.

28 Singh A, Yadav S. Microneedling: advances and widening horizons. Indian Dermatol Online J. 2016;7:244–254.

29 Asif M, Kanodia S, Singh K. Combined autologous platelet-rich plasma with microneedling verses microneedling with distilled water in the treatment of atrophic acne scars: a concurrent split-face study. J Cosmet Dermatol. 2016;15:434–443.

30 Dhurat R, Sukesh M, Avhad G, et al. A randomized evaluator blinded study of effect of microneedling in androgenetic alopecia: a pilot study. Int J Trichol. 2013;5:6–11.

31 Kumar MK, Inamadar AC, Palit A. A randomized controlled single-observer blinded study to determine the efficacy of topical minoxidil plus microneedling versus topical minoxidil alone in the treatment of androgenetic alopecia. J Cutan Aesthet Surg. 2018;11:211–216.

32 Messenger AG, Rundegren J. Minoxidil: mechanisms of action on hair growth. Br J Dermatol. 2004;150:186–194.

33 Pekmezci E, Turkoglu M, Gokalp H, et al. Minoxidil downregulates interleukin-1 alpha gene expression in HaCaT cells. Int J Trichol. 2018;10:108–112.

34 Alkhalifah A, Alsantali A, Wang E, et al. Alopecia areata update: part II. Treatment. J Am Acad Dermatol. 2010;62:191–202.

35 Gupta A, Aggarwal G, Singla S, Arora R. Transfersomes: A Novel Vesicular Carrier for Enhanced Transdermal Delivery of Sertraline: Development, Characterization, and Performance Evaluation. Sci Pharm. 2012;80(4):1061–1080.

36 Lynch MD, Bashir S. Applications of platelet-rich plasma in dermatology: A critical appraisal of the literature. J Dermatolog Treat. 2016;27(3):285–289. doi:10.3109/09546 634.2015.1094178

37 Blair P, Flaumenhaft R. Platelet α-granules: basic biology and clinical correlates. Blood Rev. 2009;23:177–189.

38 Eppley BL, Woodell JE, Higgins J. Platelet Quantification and Growth Factor Analysis from Platelet-Rich Plasma: Implications for Wound Healing, Plastic and Reconstructive Surgery: November 2004, Volume 114, Issue 6, pp1502–1508.

39 Trink A, Sorbellini E, Bezzola P, et al. A randomized, double-blind, placebo- and active-controlled, half-head study to evaluate the effects of platelet-rich plasma on alopecia areata. Br J Dermatol. 2013;169(3):690–694.

Index

Note: Page numbers in *italic* refer to figures, page numbers in **bold** refer to tables.

Microneedling: Global Perspectives in Aesthetic Medicine, First Edition.
Edited by Elizabeth Bahar Houshmand.
© 2021 John Wiley & Sons Ltd. Published 2021 by John Wiley & Sons Ltd.